THE SPEECH OF
HEARING-IMPAIRED
CHILDREN

To Maria

ANDREAS MARKIDES

The speech of hearing-impaired children

Manchester University Press

Published by Manchester University Press
Oxford Road, Manchester M13 9PL
and 51 Washington St, Dover
New Hampshire 03820, USA

British Library cataloguing in publication data

Markides, Andreas
    The speech of hearing-impaired children.
    1. Hearing disorders in children
    2. Children language
    I. Title
    401′.9   RF219.5.C45

ISBN 0-7190-0915-4
ISBN 0-7190-0951-0 Pbk

*Library of Congress cataloging in
publication data
Applied for*

Printed in Great Britain
at the Alden Press, Oxford

CONTENTS

FOREWORD

The teaching of speech to deaf children provides an exciting and challenging task to teachers of the deaf. It certainly did to me when I began to try to do this more than forty-five years ago, and it has done so in Britain, as Dr Markides explains, for well over three hundred years. It therefore gives me much pleasure to introduce this fresh contribution to the field especially as the author has effectively combined an academic study of the subject with practical procedures.

Despite the length of time during which the teaching of speech has been practised, however, the end-products have not always reached the hoped-for standards. When Charles Sheriff (Thomas Braidwood's first pupil in 1760) spoke, a contemporary witness reported, it was 'harsh and grating to the ear' and a large number of people 'could never understand a single sentence of Mr. Sheriff's'. In his National Survey of Speech Intelligibility of 1981, Dr Markides found that the speech of 38% of the pupils in schools for the deaf was very poor, and only 40% attained an acceptable level. Although it would therefore hardly be true to say that we have not come very far in the intervening period, we have certainly not come as far as we would have wished, even allowing for the formidable nature of the task.

In the opening chapter Dr Markides considers the history of developments in the teaching of speech. He documents carefully the lessons to be learned from these past methodologies and, in relation to the current opposition of views about intervention or non-intervention in speech development, takes the view, with which I must agree, that it is unwise to abandon methods and procedures that have been successful when applied with insight and care in favour of an unquestioning acceptance of new theories which have not yet proved that they are superior.

Starting from a careful analysis of speech errors Dr Markides provides us with much up-to-date information, both from his own and other relevant researches, about the intelligibility of deaf children's speech. In particular, the National Survey, referred to above, provides information concerning the present position which will be invaluable to all those concerned with the education of hearing-impaired children. Since we now know so much more about factors that make for greater intelligibility and can capitalise on this in our teaching, it is evident that improvements should be able to be made and this book has much to offer on the basic principles, objectives and strategies that will enable a competent teacher to meet the needs of individual children.

This is a timely book. There is currently a considerable body of opinion in this country and elsewhere in favour of using what is described as 'total communication' in the education of deaf children and, whilst the supporters of this method claim to include the use of hearing aids and the teaching of speech amongst the ingredients of a total approach, there seems to be a large element of manualism in the classrooms where the system is employed. This seems odd when current attitudes towards handicapped people emphasise a greater integration into normal society and when the most recent Education Act is aiming at a marked increase in the assimilation of hearing-impaired children into ordinary schools and classes. One might assume that this could best come about by the improvement, wherever possible, in normal communication skills amongst deaf children. These skills would be, from the receptive angle, the use of residual hearing, lipreading and reading: from the expressive side they would be speech and writing. On this basis, and in accordance with the philosophy outlined above, Dr Markides has set out a 'Delivery System' which I believe would go a very long way towards bringing deaf children nearer the goal of integration. The task of teachers is clear: they must master the facts, determine their objectives and actively help children to acquire the appropriate skills. This book will help them to do all of these things.

T. J. WATSON

PREFACE

This book is about the speech of hearing-impaired children. It looks critically at the speech abilities of such children and on the basis of past practices, recent research findings and experience puts forward a model or framework for the teaching of speech. In detail the book is divided into three parts.

Part I deals with the historical developments and research evidence regarding the teaching of speech. It consists of two chapters. Chapter 1 describes and discusses the historical developments in the teaching of speech to hearing-impaired people from ancient times right down to the present day and Chapter 2 presents the major studies into the speech of hearing-impaired children.

Part II deals with the speech attainments and speech disorders of hearing-impaired children. It consists of five chapters. Chapter 3 presents the articulatory features of the speech of hearing-impaired children and Chapter 4 presents the prosodic features. Chapter 5 deals with overall speech intelligibility, Chapter 6 deals with speech assessment procedures, and Chapter 7 presents and discusses the findings of a national survey into the speech intelligibility of hearing-impaired children.

The purpose of Part III is to integrate the information presented in the previous chapters into a cohesive policy or approach regarding the teaching of speech to hearing-impaired children. It presents the basic principles, objectives and strategies emerging and considers briefly normal speech development and normal speech perceptual processes. In this context knowledge of normal speech development is essential mainly because it forms the foundation on which the principles, objectives and strategies relating to the hearing-impaired children are based, provided of course, that in the process of formulating such principles, due consideration is also given to the limitations and difficulties brought about as a result of deafness. This section consists of three chapters. Chapter 8 deals with normal speech development and normal speech perceptual processes. Chapter 9 deals with the effects of hearing impairment on speech development and with the avenues and procedures available to ameliorate these effects. Chapter 10 presents the basic principles, objectives and strategies recommended in the teaching of speech to hearing-impaired children.

The book concludes with a brief statement emphasising research needs and practical developments.

This book has been written with the needs of the professional in mind – teachers of the deaf, speech therapists, linguists, phoneticians, audiologists, research workers, students in training, and others. Parents of hearing-impaired children may find some of the technical terms used rather difficult to understand but the basic concepts discussed are presented succinctly and are very easy to follow. I believe that both professionals and parents will find this book useful.

ANDREAS MARKIDES

ACKNOWLEDGEMENTS

I would like to extend my gratitude and appreciation to my wife, children, family and friends for the constant support, encouragement and understanding they have given me throughout the preparation of this book.

I am especially grateful to the hundreds of teachers of the deaf throughout the country who so willingly cooperated with my national survey on speech intelligibility. Their response to my request to participate was overwhelming and immediate and I appreciate this very much indeed.

Many others responded to my needs willingly and unselfishly to provide support and information at a moment's notice.

The actual computing of the data contained in this book took a considerable time and I am particularly grateful to Diane McCool for all her help and perseverance. Sandra Roe and Wendy Meakin illustrated the figures; and Tinna Quinn typed the entire manuscript – all my colleagues worked hard and diligently and I am grateful to them for their contribution.

PART I

Historical and research base

Those who do not learn from the past are condemned to relive it.

George Santayana

CHAPTER ONE

The teaching of speech: historical developments

Deafness presents a wide diversity of problems, the solution of which has attracted the active interest not only of educational and medical people but also of philosophers, scientists, priests, lawyers and others. A comprehensive history of the endeavours of these people to educate the deaf has yet to be written. This chapter brings together a small aspect of that history. It describes those particular developments relating to the teaching of speech to deaf children throughout the ages, from ancient times right down to the present period.

FROM ANCIENT TIMES TO THE SIXTEENTH CENTURY

The civil status of the deaf was moulded and controlled for nearly two thousand years by a misconception regarding the origins of speech. This misconception came about as a result of a very passionate and extensive philosophical debate as to whether speech was of divine or human origin. Plato wrote extensively on this and so did successive generations of linguistic researchers. The arguments were bitter and long, and in retrospect it seems that each researcher favoured the solution most compatible with his own personal point of view. Unfortunately throughout ancient times and also during the Middle Ages the theory of the divine origin of speech was almost universally accepted, so much so that the story of the Tower of Babel was not considered as merely a parable.

The theory of the divine origin of speech coupled with Aristotle's teachings that nothing can exist in the human mind that has not been received through the senses (*nihil est in intellectu, quin prius fuerit in sensu* – History of Animals) had a profound effect on the way deaf people were perceived and treated by important sections of society such as the established church, the legislature and medicine.

The church adhered to the theory that speech was of divine origin, and therefore, naturally considered that to try to teach the deaf to speak was blasphemous. If speech was forbidden them then that was God's will and no attempt should be made to change it. Even as late as the eighteenth century Abbé de l'Épée had to fight against this argument, for the accusation hurled against him by his fellow priests that his entire venture in teaching the deaf to speak was contrary to God's will, was a very serious matter. The church also considered the ears to be the '*instrumentum disciplinae*', the '*porta mentis*', and since, in the theological point of view, man acquired faith only by hearing the doctrinal teaching, a deaf person could not participate in religion. St Paul's dictum in the Epistle to the Romans (x, 17) 'faith is obtained through hearing' was quoted time and again in support of this dogma and eventually it was taken to mean that the deaf were deprived of salvation. Of course St Paul's '*fides ex auditu*' was purely a figure of speech, meaning those people who wished to hear and did not reject the word of God. But even as early as the fourth century, St Augustine in his treatise against the Pelasgians took it literally and interpreted it to mean that, according to Paul, faith had been denied to the deaf and therefore they should not be educated because God had branded them as a punishment to sinful parents. This erroneous interpretation of the epistle gained increasing acceptance and by the end of the sixteenth century a commentator even took St Augustine's explanation as being the original text (Werner, 1932). Eventually this attitude brought about a violent dispute between the Catholic and Protestant churches. In this dispute Luther, contrary to the teachings of the Catholic Church, took the point of view that deaf people who were not insane should not be denied religion and should even be allowed to participate in Holy Communion.

In legislature also the deaf were heavily discriminated against. The ancient Roman law placed the deaf and dumb in the same category as imbeciles and therefore ineducable. Consequently a deaf and dumb person could not in law be granted a fully responsible role in society. Pre-Justinian jurisprudence improved slightly on this but still the deaf and dumb were not allowed to participate in any legal business that required speech. The greatest difficulty here was the question of whether deaf-mutes were capable of making a will and of inheriting and passing on property. This problem came to a head in Spain in the sixteenth century when a number of aristocratic families with enormous wealth discovered that some of their sons and daughters were deaf. Property, inheritance and prestige were at stake. Action was needed and action was taken. The aristocratic families knew of the successes of Pedro Ponce in teaching the deaf to speak. They quickly arranged for gifted teachers to teach their children to speak. The results were remarkable and their hired lawyers argued (Lasso, 1550) that deaf-mutes who had learned to speak could no longer be called deaf-mutes and from the legal point of view they should not be treated as such and should be allowed to inherit family property. The amount of legal argument on this subject was vast and continued right up to the beginning of the nineteenth century. Old arguments concerning the impossibility of teaching deaf-mutes to speak were rekindled and they were exactly the same as those put forward in medical literature. Their net effect was to impede rather than promote progress. Legislation concerning deaf-mutes remained unchanged until the middle of the eighteenth century when the old laws were finally outstripped by actual practice.

One would have expected medical theory and practice to pioneer change and to bring about progress in the understanding and treatment of deafness. Far from it. Medical theory and practice for centuries failed to appreciate the consequential connection between deafness and dumbness. It was thought that dumbness was caused by damage to the nerves controlling the movements of the tongue and thus the deaf were unable to move their tongues in order to articulate. This misconception stemmed primarily from the writings of Hippocrates (not Aristotle as often quoted) who stated that the tongue alone effects articulation. Thus if the tongue movements are impeded by any cause then it is impossible to speak. Unfortunately Hippocrates cited as evidence of this congenitally deaf people who could not speak. Even when it had been proved in practice that a deaf-mute could be taught to speak (late sixteenth century), the doctors tried to prove anatomically that this could not have been so and that the deaf-mutes who had been successfully taught to speak were not really deaf-mutes but a special type whose lingual nerves remained undamaged.

By asserting that a form of paralysis of the tongue existed in cases of deafness and dumbness, medicine did a great disservice to the deaf. It effectively condemned to failure any attempt to teach the deaf to speak. Legislation and the church also did a great disservice to the deaf by explicitly laying down the principle that deaf-mutes could not be educated and thus establishing the reasons by which the deaf were in general cut off from civil life.

THE DISCOVERY OF SPEECH TEACHING

The first attempt to teach speech to a deaf-mute was attributed to the Bishop of Hagulstad (later on called St John of Beverley). The story of the bishop and the deaf and dumb youth was related by the Venerable Bede (AD 674–735) who was inclined to view the matter as more a miracle than a natural consequence of education. A similar case was reported nearly eight centuries afterwards by Rudolf Agricola, although in this instance the teacher involved was not mentioned. There is no doubt, however, that speech teaching as such was discovered in Spain in the sixteenth century.

The three pioneers who were principally involved in this were Pedro Ponce de León (1529–84), Manuel Ramirez de Cárrion (1579–1652) and Juan Martin Pablo Bonet (1570–1629). According to Kröhnert (1966) the first was the inventor, the second the real expert and the third the theorist.

Pedro Ponce was a Benedictine monk who was living in Spain in the San Salvador de Ona Monastery, near Burgos. By chance he met two deaf and dumb boys of aristocratic origin who were placed in the custody of the monastery. The two boys became very closely attached to Brother Pedro Ponce, who decided to teach them the 'comforts of religious belief' and in doing so he found a way of communicating with them. As far as we know, he first tried only written communication but later on he investigated whether his pupils could also produce speech. The results were encouraging. Don Pedro, the younger of his two pupils, benefited so much from his teacher's training

> that, having no more hearing than a stone, he could talk, although admittedly with a severe stutter. He wrote with a good style, read and understood Italian and Latin books and could discuss any subject whatsoever . . . his speech was somewhat clumsy but the subtlety of his argument compensated for this drawback. [Werner, 1932]

No written documentation of Ponce's methods survived. According to the chronicler Ambrosio de Morales (1575), quoted by Arnold (1888), Don Pedro described his master's methods as follows:

> You see, when I was young and as ignorant as a stone, I began to learn to write and first of all I wrote the names of objects which my teacher showed me. Then I wrote all the Spanish words in a book which was provided me for this purpose. Then, with God's help. I began to spell out and speak as loudly as I could, although a great deal of spittle came from my mouth. Afterwards I began to read stories so that in ten years I had read stories from all over the world. Then I learned Latin. This all happened by God's great grace without which nothing can succeed . . .

Apart from these two sons of the Velasco family, Ponce educated a whole series of other deaf-mutes, again exclusively drawn from aristocratic families – the two Velasco sisters, the son of the senior judge of Aragon, the sons of the Constable of Castile and others. He taught them to speak, read, write, calculate, pray, assist at mass, know the creed and confess orally. He taught some to understand Latin, Greek and Italian. His results were acclaimed by the public as one of the greatest miracles that had ever happened in the world. The medical fraternity, however, received Ponce's successes in teaching the deaf to speak with great scepticism. At best it was thought that Ponce had, by the grace of God, been given a purely personal, almost miraculous talent for teaching speech to deaf-mutes like Christ's curing of the dumb. At worst Ponce's successes were dismissed as irrelevant and without any foundation.

Pedro Ponce lived to a good old age and died a very famous man in 1584. His epitaph read 'Here lies the venerable Father Pedro Ponce, who deserves to be eternally remembered for his gift, given him by God, for making the dumb speak . . .'

The second of the three pioneers was Manuel Ramirez de Cárrion, a school teacher by profession and as far as we know a teacher of both hearing and deaf pupils. His expertise with deaf pupils was quickly seized upon by the Spanish aristocracy. Most probably it was Ramirez who invented speech training but unfortunately he was not given proper recognition for this until 1924 when Navarro-Tomas published his well documented work. Prior to this, Ramirez was cruelly misjudged and was considered either as a fraud or as a person of minor importance. His more illustrious contemporary and acquaintance, Juan Pablo Bonet, who probably borrowed most of his ideas on deaf education from Ramirez, totally eclipsed him in reputation. According to Juan Batista Morales (quoted by Arnold, 1888) it was Ramirez de Cárrion who used extensively what we now call the phonic method of reading, by which the individual letters of the alphabet are presented in their actual spoken values. By using this method Ramirez claimed that he could teach intelligent people to both read and write within two weeks and also following the same method he could teach deaf people to speak. Ramirez's claims were greatly undermined by Bonet who stated in his book, published in 1620, that it was he who was the first to invent the simplification of the alphabet and the reduction of the individual letters to their sound elements as a method for teaching deaf people to speak.

Juan Pablo Martin Bonet was born an aristocrat in Torres de Berrelen towards the last quarter of the sixteenth century. Contrary to popular belief Bonet was not a teacher of the deaf but a soldier, a man of letters and a politician. He filled various important positions in the service of King Philip including that of secretary to the Constable of Castile. Bonet came to know the Velasco family very well and volunteered to find out how help could be obtained for one of the boys, Luis de Velasco, who was deaf. His search led him to Ramirez de Cárrion who was at the time engaged in teaching speech to the deaf Marquis de Priego. Ramirez de Cárrion took on the job of educating the young Luis. He taught him for four years with remarkable success and in 1619 Ramirez returned to his previous appointment with the Marquis de Priego. A year after this, Bonet, who was not involved with the education of the deaf boy but most probably was able to observe and discuss in detail Ramirez's methods, published the first book of deaf education, entitled *Simplification of the Letters of the Alphabet and Method of Teaching Deaf-Mutes to Speak* (Bonet, 1620).

Nowhere in his book did Bonet make any reference to the work of Ponce de Léon or Ramirez de Cárrion. He presented himself as the sole originator of the method he described and this, most probably, contributed significantly in bringing upon himself the accusation of being a plagiarist and a fraud.

His book was divided into two parts. In the first part he presented a description of the phonetic qualities of the letters of the alphabet and in the second part he described in detail his method of teaching the deaf to speak.

In detail Bonet's speech training method was as follows. First of all the deaf pupil should practise writing the individual letters of the alphabet. Then the one-handed manual alphabet should be introduced and the pupil given very basic and extensive training in it. Only when the pupil had a basic knowledge of writing and of the hand alphabet should the teacher go on and introduce speech training. During speech teaching Bonet recommended that the teacher and pupil should be left alone because the task was considered to require a great deal of attention and concentration. The teacher was advised to place himself in a good light so that the pupil could obtain a clear view of his mouth. Then the teacher should begin by teaching the vowels before dealing with the consonants. He suggested the making of a tongue out of leather in order to demonstrate its position when articulating the various sounds. Then the deaf pupil was taught syllables, followed by simple monosyllabic words, preferably of objects at hand that could be pointed at for association purposes. Upon acquiring a basic vocabulary the deaf pupil was then taught the Spanish language in well documented grammatical steps which were supplemented with extensive reading. Bonet did not emphasise the need for lipreading.

The influence of the Spanish pioneers spread throughout Europe including the United Kingdom. No attempt will be made in this chapter to describe in detail the relevant developments in mainland Europe – their influence on the British scene, however, will be traced and documented.

BRITISH DEVELOPMENTS

SEVENTEENTH CENTURY

The Spanish connection and subsequent developments

The Spanish connection with the British scene came about when Luis de Velasco, the deaf boy whom we have already met as a pupil of Ramirez de Cárrion, encountered Prince Charles of England in the court of King Philip in 1623. Prince Charles was most impressed with the linguistic and social achievements of the young deaf aristocrat. So were his companions, among whom was Sir Kenelme Digby. On his return to England Digby wrote a book in which he described Luis de Velasco as follows:

> . . . so deaf that if a gun were shot off close to his eare he could not heare it, and consequently he was dumb . . . there was a priest [most probably he refers to Bonet!] who . . . after strange patience, constancy, and paines, he brought the young lord to speak as distinctly as any man soever; and to understand so perfectly what others said that he would not lose a word in a whole day's conversation . . . It is true, one great misbecomingness he was apt to fall into, whiles he spoke: which was an uncertainty in the tone of his voice; for not hearing the sound he made when he spoke, he could not steadily governe the pitch of his voyce, but it would be sometimes higher, sometimes lower though for the most part, what he delivered together, he ended in the same key as he began it.

In Britain the honour of being the first to write extensively on the subject of deafness goes to John Bulwer. Surprisingly we have very little information about Bulwer's life. We know that he was a physician, and that most of his writings have survived but neither the date of his birth nor his death are known. He was certainly aware of Digby's account of the achievements of Luis de Velasco and, most probably, it was through reading this account that he came to know of Bonet's work. In 1648 he published *Philocophus, or the Deafe and Dumbe Man's Friend*. In this he dealt with the principles of teaching speech and language to the deaf. Bulwer, contrary to the teachings of the Spanish pioneers, made lipreading or 'ocular audition', as Digby referred to it, the *sine qua non* of his teaching system.

'Exhibiting the philosophical verity of that subtile art, which may enable one (born deaf and dumb) with an observant eye, to hear what any man speaks by the moving of his lips . . . and thence learn to speak with his tongue.' The first step, however, was writing and the hand alphabet. In addition to this he advocated that gesture be used for purposes of instruction. It is true that, like the Spanish pioneers, his interest in deafness was aroused by one or two 'gentlemen' who were deaf and 'although proficient in the use of signs and the manual alphabet, desired to acquire speech'. Bulwer, however, did not restrict himself to the philosophy of merely teaching individual deaf-mutes. He was the first person in Europe to suggest and pursue the founding of an 'Academy for deaf-mutes'. Unfortunately, he has never been given the proper credit he deserves for this endeavour. Indeed, his book was most probably written with the express intention of publicising his idea of an academy.

> I began in idea, to conceive the modell of a new Academie which might be erected in favour of those, who are in your condition, to wit originally deafe

and dumbe, for which edifice and Gymnasium haveing provided all kinde of materials requisite I soon perceived by falling into discourse with some rationall men about such a disigne, that the attempt seemed so paradoxi- call, prodigious and hyperbolicall, that it did rather amuse than satisfie their understandings, insomuch as they tooke the tearmes and expressions this art justly usurpes for insufferable violations of their reason, which they professed, they must renounce before they could have faith to credit such an undertaking.

Bulwer's idea for the establishment of an actual institution or academy for deaf-mutes did not reach fruition. Most probably this was due, not only to the lack of finance and understanding among influential people, but also to the fact that Bulwer was basically a theoretician and a visionary without any practical experience in this field. Not long after Bulwer, however, new developments, especially in the field of phonetics, coupled with the sustained influence of the three Spanish pioneers, gave new impetus to the education of deaf-mutes. In Britain the main personality associated with these developments was John Wallis.

Wallis (1616–1703) was a clergyman and mathematician who became professor of geometry at the University of Oxford. In 1653 he published his *Grammatica Lingua Anglicanae*. In this book he included a chapter on speech (*De Loquela*) in which he analysed and described the formation of all the different sounds in the English language. He classified vowels according to their position and manner of articulation and noted the effects of the position or shape of the speech organs on the production of vowels. He divided the consonants into two classes – open and closed, and he described the articulation of the affricates and the semi-vowels very accurately. He claimed to have been the first to attempt a complete scientific analysis of speech and in a letter addressed to Dr Thomas Smith and published in 1725 he described his speech teaching method as follows: 'In pursuance of this, I thought it very possible to teach a deaf person to speak, by directing him, so to apply the organs of speech, as the sound of each letter required.' There is no doubt that Wallis was a very important man but there is nothing original in his speech teaching method. William Holder (1669), another eminent clergyman who had practical experience in the teaching of speech, accused Wallis of being an impostor and a plagiarist. With hindsight, the same accusation can be levelled against Wallis with regard to his method of teaching language to the deaf and dumb. Wallis's language scheme was remarkably similar to that put forward by Dalgarno in 1680 in his *Didascalocophus*. Wallis knew of Dalgarno's work but he failed even to mention it, let alone acknowledge it. In retrospect it seems that it was Dalgarno, the shrewd Scotsman, who was the true originator of the ideas put forward by Wallis and in view of this the honour of being the father of deaf education in Great Britain should go to Dalgarno and not to Wallis as hitherto.

EIGHTEENTH CENTURY

Braidwood's academy and European developments

During the first half of the eighteenth century very little progress was made in the education of the deaf in Britain. The only name that has come down to us in this connection is that of Henry Baker (1698–1774), a Londoner, who was a well known naturalist and poet. He had excellent connections with the nobility and had, for a period of time, attempted to teach several deaf pupils with aristocratic backgrounds. From all we know his results were impressive but unfortunately owing to his pathological secretiveness, nothing of his methods has survived. Another person who later on had an enormous influence on deaf education in Britain was John Conrad Amman (1669–1724). Amman was a medical man from Switzerland who later on, because of religious persecution, settled in Holland. His book *Surdus Loquens* (The speaking deaf) was first published in 1692 and was immediately translated into English. In this book, which was later revised and extended under the title *Dissertatio de Loquela*, he described his method of teaching deaf-mutes to speak as follows. He first satisfied himself that the pupil 'was of a quick and docile disposition, neither too young nor too old, but verging on youth, between eight and fifteen years of age and that his organs of speech were perfect'. Then he would 'get him to produce a clear emission of the voice and have the power of controlling it'. At the outset he put great stress on the value of touch, as enabling the deaf to have an intuitive perception of sounds which he called 'the great mystery of the art, and is, if it is right so to speak, the hearing of the deaf, or at all events what is analogous to it'. The next step involved the teaching of the pupil to pronounce first the vowels, then the semi-vowels and next the consonants, at the same time making him repeat and write them from dictation, or recite from the written forms until, by constant repetition, the association between speech and writing was firmly established. To assist the scholar a mirror was used. Amman regarded the pronunciation of the vowels as a 'critical exercise' and he considered the consonants as comparatively easy to articulate. His next step was the combining of the sounds learned, proceeding to the pronunciation of syllables and words, beginning with the easiest. Later, he made his pupils read a book, which he closed at the end of each line; then, securing their attention, pronounced the words which they repeated after him. Thus Amman closely associated reading with speaking. In lipreading he encouraged his pupils to lipread not only himself but also one another too (Farrar, 1923).

By the middle of the eighteenth century a considerable amount of groundwork had already been done both in mainland Europe and in Britain. Speech sounds had been analysed and described with remarkable accuracy and a practical method of teaching speech to 'deaf and dumb' children had been developed. A large number of 'deaf people' were taught to speak, but still teaching was an individual affair exclusively limited to the very few – the sons and daughters of the nobility. This was the situation inherited by Thomas Braidwood, a Scot, who in 1760 took the next logical step and established the first school for the deaf in Edinburgh.

Thomas Braidwood was born in 1715 but his early life is rather obscure. We know that he attended the University of Edinburgh and after working as an assistant in a grammar school he branched out and 'opened a school for the instruction of young men in geometry, mathematics etc' (*Gentleman's Magazine*, 1807). Later on he started his school for the deaf in 1760 with only one pupil. His teaching practices were based on the theories suggested by Wallis (Gallaudet, 1910). He continued to teach the deaf for the next twenty years and by 1780 his school had expanded to twenty pupils (all boarders) and two masters. Braidwood was very secretive about his methods of teaching and the little we now know is based on the accounts of third parties who either worked with him or came to know his school as visitors. The best account of his school is that given by Francis Green, an American, whose son was a pupil at the school.

According to Monboddo (quoted by Arnold, 1888) instruction at the school began with the teaching of speech.

> They at first only breathe strongly till they are taught that concussion and tremulous motion of the windpipe produces audible sounds. Having been taught to produce sound, the pupils were then taught to articulate the five vowels in doing which, the teacher is obliged, not only himself to use many distortions and grimaces in order to show his pupils the positions and actions of the several organs, but likewise to employ his hands to place and move their organs properly.

Green (1783) takes on the description by stating that 'When the five vowels can be distinctly sounded and discriminated then an easy monosyllable is learned as Ba, be & C . . . Suppose the learner to be perfect in pronouncing Ba; then by placing his tongue in such a position as to add T, the word BAT is formed.' Braidwood used 'a small round piece of silver of a few inches long, the size of a tobacco pipe, flattened at one end, with a ball (as large as a marble) at the other;' by means of which he manipulated the tongue of the pupils into the correct positions for the articulation of different vowels and consonants. When the pupil had learned to articulate a word correctly then the object was pointed out to him so that the association of the spoken word with the object could be established. This order of presentation, namely speech, association with object, then writing, was later on changed to writing, articulation and then association with object. Whichever order was followed, however,

'The greatest care must be taken never to proceed to a new sound until the preceding has become familiar.' (Watson, 1809).

The next stage involved the expansion of the pupil's vocabulary – naming visible objects and their qualities, including parts of the body, dress, articles of furniture, animals. Pronouns and verbs were then introduced leading on to the construction of simple sentences, longer sentences, etc.

Green (1783) gave the following interesting account of the achievements of his son who was then 9 years old and had received tuition from Braidwood for a period of 15 months:

> The child eagerly advanced and addressed me with a distinct salutation of speech. He also made several enquiries in short sentences: I then delivered him a letter from his sister which he read so as to be understood; he accompanied many of the words as he pronounced them with proper gestures significant of their meaning . . . He could at that time repeat the Lord's prayer very properly . . .

Many other visitors to the school were highly impressed. It seems that Braidwood's successes were considerable. His pupils, within a period of only five years' tuition, were reasonably educated; they could read and write, their lipreading was good and they could communicate through speaking. The standards achieved were high and the reputation of Braidwood and his academy spread all over the country and abroad.

In 1783 Braidwood closed his Edinburgh academy and moved south and established a new school at Hackney. His work stimulated public interest and in 1792 we see the establishment of the first public institution for the deaf in the UK, the Old Kent Road Asylum for the Deaf and Dumb, with Braidwood's nephew, Joseph Watson, as principal.

Thomas Braidwood's original contribution to the teaching of speech was limited. We know from his nephew's writings (Watson, 1809) that his methods were based upon Wallis and that he followed a combined approach rather than the pure oralism of the German school. This, however, must not be allowed to detract from the great achievements of this pioneer. His was the initiative to set up the first school for the deaf in Britain, his was the inspiration that more similar institutions should be founded and above all, his was the teaching ability that showed that the deaf could achieve reasonable oral skills.

Despite all his achievements, Braidwood has not always been well remembered, especially by the Americans. The reasons for this stem from two sources, both of them intimately connected with developments in deaf education in the USA.

The first source of discontent related to Thomas Hopkins Gallaudet, an American, who was sent to Britain to study the oral method. The Braidwoods refused to divulge their method to him. As a result of this refusal Gallaudet went to France and became closely associated with the French method (the manual method) of teaching the deaf. On his return to the USA he, of course, introduced the manual methodologies of the French, instead of the predominantly oral method of Braidwood as originally intended. Although it is easy to blame the Braidwood family for this it must be noted that Gallaudet himself had a reputation for obstinacy which made him very difficult to get along with (Berger, 1972).

The second source of discontent related to John Braidwood, grandson of Thomas Braidwood, who was invited to open the first American school for the deaf at Baltimore. John Braidwood had an unfortunate start. He went to the USA in 1812 in the middle of an Anglo-American war. This, coupled with his incompetency and abrasive character, did not endear him or his family to the Americans. John Braidwood's two attempts to establish a school for the deaf in the USA met with total disaster.

The combined effects of these two sources of discontent virtually guaranteed the establishment and growth of the manual system in the USA to the neglect of the teaching of speeech to hearing-impaired children for a period of nearly a century. Later on in this chapter the enormously important American contribution to the teaching of speech will be presented, but meanwhile it is essential to describe contemporary European developments, mainly because it is primarily these developments that eventually had the greatest influence on the British scene.

During the second half of the eighteenth century in continental Europe, especially in France and Germany, the following developments were taking place.

In France Abbé de l'Epée was the first one to conceive the idea of popular education for all deaf children, including those of the poorest parents. De l'Epée, at first, taught speech in association with gesture and writing. He described his methods of teaching speech as follows:

> When I am about to teach a deaf and dumb person to pronounce, I begin with making him wash his hands thoroughly clean. This done, I trace an /A/ upon the table, 'and taking his hand, I introduce his fourth or little finger, as far as the second joint, into my mouth, after which I pronounce strongly an /A/ making him observe that my tongue lies still. [Arnold, 1888]

Later the Abbé, owing to pressure of work, abandoned the teaching of speech and concentrated his teaching exclusively on methodical signs, thus heralding a tradition of silent education for deaf children. We have no evidence as to whether de l'Epée's methods were known to Thomas Braidwood. Whatever the case may be, however, the Scotsman's work does not exhibit any traces of French influence.

Abbé de l'Epée's manual methods were heavily criticised by Samuel Heinicke (1727–90), a German organist and schoolmaster who founded the first German school for the deaf in 1778. Heinicke was greatly inspired and influenced by Johann Conrad Amman's *Surdus Loquens* and he developed the German method (oral method) as opposed to the French method (manual method) of Abbé de l'Epée. Thus began the controversy which still continues unabated between the 'manualists' on the one hand and the 'oralists' on the other.

Heinicke's method of teaching speech still remains a mystery. According to Arnold (1888), he began, like other educators of the deaf, by teaching written language first and speech afterwards but later came to believe that deaf children should be taught spoken before written language. He was of the opinion that the deaf should be taught 'as nature teaches the hearing' but the following quotation relating to his method of teaching the articulation of vowels reveals that perhaps he did not put into effect what he himself preached. 'He would give his pupils pure water for /a/, wormwood for /e/, vinegar for /i/, olive oil for /u/, the better to fix these sounds in memory.'

NINETEENTH CENTURY

Flight from speech teaching

Following the death of Thomas Braidwood in 1806 the teaching of speech in the United Kingdom declined very rapidly and eventually disappeared almost completely. It is true that for a period of 118 years (up to 1878) the headship of one or other of Britain's asylums and institutions for the deaf had been in the hands of a member of the Braidwood family. Unfortunately, however, the Braidwood name by itself was not sufficient to guarantee the continuation of speech teaching. The grandsons and nephews who followed and made up the Braidwood dynasty, simply did not prove to be as good as the grand old man.

The first half of the nineteenth century saw the establishment of asylums and institutions for the deaf and dumb in urban areas of the United Kingdom, such as Edinburgh, Aberdeen, Glasgow, Birmingham, Manchester, Liverpool, Doncaster, Brighton, Exeter, Bristol, Aberystwyth. This expansion came about mainly as a result of the endeavours of humanitarians who considered it their religious duty to provide 'places of refuge from a cruel and unsympathetic world' where the handicapped, the destitute and of course the poor should be taught to live upright and industrious lives in the position it had pleased God to place them!

The method of instruction followed in these 'schools' for the deaf was exclusively manual and the protagonist for this was Louis du Puget, a Swiss who was an ardent supporter of the methods of Abbé de l'Epée. He was appointed to the headship of the General Institution for the Instruction of the Deaf and Dumbe Children in Birmingham in 1825.

It is true that during this period there were one or two isolated attempts to teach speech but they were without success. For example, John Anderson, during his headship of the Glasgow institution, devised a model of the human speech mechanism which could be used to demonstrate the different positions required to articulate different sounds. This, however, was of no practical use and it was on show mainly to impress visitors. Also Arnold in the 1840s whilst a young teacher in the deaf institution in Liverpool (Arnold, 1888) reported that a certain amount of articulatory work (speech teaching) was attempted but without any success.

As stated, the death of Thomas Braidwood brought about a sharp decline in his partly oral methods of teaching the deaf. Within a decade of his death speech teaching in the United Kingdom was almost abandoned and so it remained for another six to seven decades.

Teaching of speech in mainland Europe

Meanwhile in Europe, especially in the German-speaking countries, Heinicke's oral methods survived and expanded mainly because of the endeavours and achievements of a few outstanding teachers of the deaf, especially Johann Baptist Graser (1766–1841), Friedrich Moritz Hill (1805–75), David Hirsch (1813–95) and Johannes Vatter (1842–1916).

Vatter is not very well known in the English-speaking world, but in Germany is still regarded as one of the most successful teachers of deaf children who has ever lived. According to Löwe (1980), Vatter was the chief exponent of the 'Association Phoneme Method' in the teaching of speech, as practised later on by Mildred McGinnis at the Central Institute for the Deaf in St Louis and only recently again recommended by Calvert and Silverman (1975). Vatter believed that it is only in a continually speaking environment that deaf children learn to connect their thoughts, feelings and ideas with the spoken word. In his book, published in 1875, he emphasised the direct association of oral language and avoidance of signs and written words. He most probably subscribed to the view, however, that tactile–kinaesthetic cues should be allowed to function in the teaching of speech and that writing could be introduced after speech had become the 'form of thinking' of the child.

Graser was the first to establish and provide education for deaf children in an ordinary school. It is only fair to mention here, however, that the first person to advocate this was a Briton John Arrowsmith in 1819 (quoted by Arnold, 1888). Graser's system, referred to as 'the generalization of the education of deaf children' did not have much chance to succeed mainly because the teacher/pupil ratio in German schools at the beginning of the nineteenth century was 1 to 80 and therefore not enough time could be spared for the slow learning deaf child. Anyway it shows that 'integration policies', which at present are considered to be the latest developments in deaf education, are not so modern after all. In reality, quite a large number of teachers of the deaf in most European countries, during the last two centuries, were advocating the desirability of educating deaf pupils in local ordinary schools where they could live at home and interact with their hearing peers (Werner, 1932; Löwe, 1980).

Graser's philosophies inspired Friedrich Moritz Hill, who later on proved to be one of the most influential and gifted teachers of the deaf (Reuschert, 1905). He studied under the famous Heinrich Pestalozzi and embraced his 'mother method' of teaching. Moritz Hill's guidelines can be summarised in the sentence: 'Teaching of spoken language is in everything.' He wanted deaf children to be introduced to language by the 'natural method' – that is in the same way as hearing children learn to speak, by constant daily use, associated with proper objects and actions. Therefore, speech in his opinion had to be taught before reading and writing and had to be used from the very beginning as the basis for teaching and communication. Natural gestures were not discouraged but needed to be replaced by speech as soon as possible.

Moritz Hill's influence spread throughout Europe. In particular his teachings fired the imagination of David Hirsch, the principal of the Rotterdam school for deaf children. Hirsch was a natural teacher, tremendously gifted and a man of great imagination. He sent his teachers to other countries carrying his oral inspirations to many places. As we shall soon see, two of his teachers, namely Gerrit van Asch and William van Praagh, were directly responsible for the revival of speech teaching in schools for the deaf in the United Kingdom.

Teaching of speech revived

The first signs of the revival of teaching speech to deaf children in the United Kingdom appeared in the early 1860s when Gerrit van Asch arrived at Manchester as tutor for the deaf-mute daughter of a wealthy Jewish merchant. A year or two later (1862), van Asch opened a private school for deaf children in London. The method of instruction in his school was oral, based on the 'German system'. In the same year, another private school for deaf children was opened in London by Susannah Hull. According to Hodgson (1953) her methods were purely oral.

In 1866 the Jewish school, under the patronage of Baroness Mayer de Rothschild, decided to adopt the oral method of education and for this purpose another Dutch national from the Rotterdam school for the deaf came over to help. The man in question was the young William van Praagh – a teacher totally committed to oralism. His oral methods proved so successful that in 1871 an Association for the Oral Instruction of the Deaf and Dumb was formed. Its aims were to publicise the oral system and to 'nationalise the oral instruction of the deaf by lipreading and articulate speech, to the rigid exclusion of the finger-alphabet and all artificial signs' and 'to train qualified teachers on this system and to maintain a normal school for instructing deaf and dumb children' (Arnold, 1888). The school and training college were opened in Fitzroy Square, London in June 1872.

By the middle of the 1870s the change in favour of teaching speech to deaf children was gathering momentum. In 1876 James Howard, the headmaster of the Yorkshire Institution for the Deaf at Doncaster, arranged for the Abbé Balestra from Italy (a convert to the 'German system') to come and instruct himself and his staff in the principles of oralism. A year later, in 1877, a conference of headmasters of institutions for the deaf was held in London. This conference, spearheaded by Richard Elliott of Margate and James Howard of Doncaster, resolved that reforms in institutions for the deaf were necessary. The next year James Watson, the last of the Braidwoods, resigned his headship at the Old Kent Road school rather than be part of the newly proposed changes.

Apart from Elliott another person was emerging to prominence at this time. He was Rev. Thomas Arnold, a successful oral teacher of the deaf and a prolific writer. Arnold's publications influenced generations of teachers of the deaf. In particular his book *A Method of Teaching the Deaf and Dumb Speech, Lip-reading, and Language* which first appeared in 1881 was adopted by the College of Teachers of the Deaf and was reprinted, with slight amendments, as recently as 1954 under the title *Arnold on the Education of the Deaf. A Manual for Teachers.*

Another influential person during this period was St John Ackers MP who had a deaf daughter. In his desire to provide for his daughter the best possible education, he visited schools for the deaf both in continental Europe and in the USA. He returned to England a firm believer in the 'German system' and he set about influencing people and events with the zeal of a missionary. He founded the 'Society for the Training of Teachers of the Deaf and the Diffusion of the German System in the United Kingdom'. In 1878 he opened a private college for training teachers of the deaf at Ealing. He publicised widely the aim of the society; he organised meetings, read papers and published pamphlets. He participated in the Royal Commission on the Condition of the Blind, and Deaf and Dumb etc. (1889) which recommended the 'pure oral method' in the education of the deaf.

The big manual 'schools' for the deaf, both in England and in continental Europe, especially in France and Italy, came under increasing public scrutiny. Their work, the living conditions of the children, their academic achievements, the calibre and training of their teachers and above all their methods of instruction were examined and found wanting. Change was demanded and change was achieved, especially following the International Congress for the Deaf, held at Milan in 1880. This congress passed the following resolutions

... considering the incontestable superiority of speech over signs in restoring the deaf-mute to society and in giving him a more perfect knowledge of the language, the Congress declares that the oral method ought to be preferred to that of signs for the education and instruction of the deaf and dumb ... and considering that the simultaneous use of speech and signs has the disadvantage of injuring speech, lip-reading and precision of ideas, declare that the pure oral method ought to be preferred ... and considering that a great number of the deaf and dumb are not receiving the benefit of instruction recommends that Governments should take the necessary steps that all the deaf and dumb may be educated. [Buxton, 1880]

Following these recommendations the official French delegate expressed his complete conversion from the manual to the oral system. So did the Italians. The English, including St John Ackers, his wife and Susannah Hull, were jubilant; the American delegation was dejected. Soon the wind of change in favour of oralism became a hurricane. In 1893 in England an Act of Parliament made the education of deaf children compulsory between the ages of 7 and 16 years. Local school boards started establishing day schools for the deaf and almost all of these schools were oral from the very beginning. Residential institutions for the deaf, in order to benefit from state financial assistance, started organising speech lessons for selected groups of deaf children.

In the USA similar developments were taking place. Manual methods of instruction, hitherto reigning supreme, were seriously challenged both in public meetings and in the courts of law. The Clarke School for the Deaf at Northampton, Massachusetts and the Lexington School for the Deaf, New York, both oral schools, were opened in the middle 1860s. Alexander Graham Bell became personally involved in the teaching of speech to deaf children. His participation during this initial and crucial period helped greatly to make the teaching of speech a success. Largely through Bell's efforts the American Association for Teaching Speech to the Deaf was founded in 1890. This association eventually developed into a national organisation of teachers and educators interested in oral instruction for the deaf.

According to Bender (1970), Bell was one of the first to advocate that deaf children begin their learning of speech by imitation of whole words, with meaning. This was contrary to the long established method of teaching speech which concentrated first on articulating single phonemes and then combining them into meaningless syllables before attempting whole words. Bell advocated a synthetic approach to the teaching of speech whereby the children were to be taught to understand whole words and sentences through lipreading and writing before attempting speech improvement.

The methods employed in the teaching of speech to deaf children, both in Europe and in the United States till the end of the nineteenth century, were essentially non-auditory. They relied mainly upon lipreading for speech reception and a combination of visual imitation and tactile and kinaesthetic training for speech production. At about the turn of the century, a new development entered into the education of the deaf which was to have far-reaching effects. Alexander Graham Bell invented the 'audiometer' and he used it to investigate the residual hearing of the pupils in schools for the deaf. His investigations were not very successful, mainly because of the low intensity of sound that could be produced with the new instrument. In the United Kingdom Dr James Kerr Love in 1893 reported that fewer than 10 per cent of the pupils in the Glasgow Institution for the Deaf were totally deaf. The rest could hear loud speech and he urged that the residual capacity to hear of the pupils in institutions for the deaf could be a decisive factor in their speech improvement (Kerr Love and Addison, 1896). Meanwhile in Europe Victor Urbantschitsch, Friedrich Bezold and Karl Kroiss were also advocating the use of residual hearing. In this context two publications need to be mentioned, the first one by Kroiss (1903) entitled *The Methodics of Auditory Education* and the second one *The Acoustic Method* by Goldstein (1939) who had worked under Urbantschitsch in Vienna before returning to the USA. Max Goldstein became a strong advocate of the importance of residual hearing. He also developed methods of making deaf children aware of sounds by using vibration through the use of touch. He worked in St Joseph's School for the Deaf, in St Louis, Missouri and in 1897 he set up a programme in acoustic stimulation whereby each child was given acoustic exercises for 15 minutes daily. These exercises, according to Goldstein (1939), brought about better speech comprehension and better speech intelligibility.

Strictly speaking the importance of using the residual hearing of deaf children in their education was realised much earlier than Urbantschitsch. It was already known in France at the time of Ernaud, Pereira, Deschamps and Perolle, and later on by Jean Gaspard Marie Itard (1775–1838), the great exponent of the unisensory approach.

TWENTIETH CENTURY TRENDS

Any survey of developments or trends regarding the teaching of speech to deaf children in the present century cannot be objective in the same sense as were the earlier sections of this chapter. The distance from events is too short, the personal involvements are too great, and the mass of relevant information is too overpowering to allow a balanced judgement as to what is permanent and what is only of passing value. A similar exercise undertaken even twenty-five years ago, when the present author entered the field of deaf education, would undoubtedly have emphasised events and methods that are now long forgotten, while overlooking advances that have since proved to be of great importance and vitality. This section will, therefore, be weighed down with as few names and details as possible and it will concentrate primarily on developments in the United Kingdom.

In spite of the unprecedented achievements of this century, most of the prominent and 'modern' traits in deaf education were actually well in evidence in the nineteenth century – the use of the residual hearing of deaf children, the training of teachers of the deaf in the oral methods of teaching, the importance of early education for deaf children, day educational provision and integration programmes, state involvement, parental involvement and of course changes in basic educational philosophy.

The first few years of the twentieth century in the United Kingdom witnessed the slow but steady (re)introduction of the teaching of speech in the old residential institutions for the deaf. During the next twenty to thirty years the pace quickened considerably in spite of the reluctance and misgivings of most headmasters.

This accelerated change was to a large extent due to the pioneer work of Dr Kerr Love in Glasgow. His researches on residual hearing convinced him that its use was of paramount importance for the education of deaf children. This led him to believe that there was a need for both early education for deaf children and also separate educational provision for those children who could talk before the onset of deafness. At his suggestion in 1908 the Glasgow School Board established the first special school for children who became deaf after learning to talk and two years afterwards they appointed the first 'peripatetic' teacher of the deaf for domiciliary work with the families of very young deaf children. This led to the establishment, in the same city, of a nursery school for deaf children in 1911. The idea caught on and the following year saw the establishment of the first public residential infant school for deaf children at the Royal School for the Deaf in Manchester with Miss I. R. Goldsack (later Lady Irene Ewing) as teacher-in-charge. This lady and her husband, the late Professor Sir Alexander Ewing, were destined to have the most remarkable influence on the education of deaf children, not only in the UK but all over the world. Their contributions will be made clear as the chapter progresses.

The teaching of speech to deaf children during this period underwent a significant change and this is best illustrated by the work of Arthur J. Story, who was headmaster of the North Staffordshire Joint Committee's Residential School for the Blind and Deaf at Stoke-on-Trent. In 1901 he published his first book entitled *Speech for the Deaf*. This book consisted primarily of 38 lessons in speech. The method put forward involved a child's learning to pronounce a particular vowel or consonant, first by itself, then in syllables and after that in words. His second book entitled *Speech, Reading and Speech for the Deaf* was published in 1915. In this book Story repudiated his earlier speech teaching methodology and wrote as follows: 'The articulation class of our earlier days with its dreary daily successions and repetitions of "a", "pa", "tha" etc; dead and meaningless to the child . . .'. He went on to suggest a synthetic and more natural approach to the teaching of speech whereby the parents were to be encouraged to participate as early as possible.

The contribution of Arthur J. Story to the teaching of speech was invaluable but it was soon eclipsed by the brilliance of G. Sibley Haycock whose influence in this area is still with us. Haycock was a successful oral teacher of the deaf. He became the principal of the training college and school at Fitzroy Square, London, and following his unsuccessful attempt in 1919 to become the first lecturer in deaf education at the University of Manchester, he went on to accept the post of superintendent of the Langside School for the Deaf, Glasgow. His lifelong interest was the teaching of speech and in 1933 he published his book entitled *The Teaching of Speech*. This book became a classic. It was reprinted 19 times, the last one as recently as 1979. Haycock's methodologies of teaching speech to deaf children were systematic and thorough. Throughout his book he emphasised both the prosodic aspects of speech (rhythm, phrasing, intonation, rate of speaking, breath control and voice quality) and the articulatory aspects of speech. He provided accurate description regarding the production of each phoneme and advocated a synthetic approach to the teaching of speech with special emphasis on the connected speech of deaf children. His method of teaching was primarily a visual method depending on lipreading and direct imitation assisted when necessary by touch and kinaesthetic sensation.

A major development which influenced the teaching of speech to deaf children in the twentieth century was the training of teachers of the deaf. From the very beginning in the UK the official training of teachers of the deaf, both at Fitzroy Square and Ealing in London and later on at the University of Manchester, was based on the oral method. In 1912 the two London colleges came together at Fitzroy Square. This amalgamation, however, was short-lived for the combined college at Fitzroy Square was soon absorbed into the Faculty of Education of the University of Manchester.

In 1919 the University of Manchester, after accepting a trust from a Lancashire cotton merchant, Sir James Jones, established a lectureship for training teachers of the deaf on the oral method of teaching (Whitton, 1956) and this in effect was the foundation of the present Department of Audiology and Education of the Deaf. The first lecturer to be appointed, and the person who made the department, was Irene Goldsack (Ewing, 1956) who later became Lady Irene Ewing. The department stayed in the hands of the Ewings for nearly half a century, until the middle 1960s, and during this period it became the focus of both national and international development and innovation in the education of deaf children. Over the years thousands of teachers of the deaf, not only from the UK but from all over the world, especially from Commonwealth countries, were trained in the department and the oral methods of the Ewings spread far and wide. In the last twenty years, however, the training of teachers of the deaf in the United Kingdom has been diversified, so much so that at present we can no longer assume that all future teachers of the deaf in the country will be trained in the oral method of teaching the deaf.

The achievements of the Ewings were enormous and they rightly deserve a unique and honoured place in the history of deaf education. Theirs was the pioneering spirit that brought about early ascertainment of deafness and widespread use of amplification in schools for the deaf. It was primarily through their teachings that the need for a variety of educational provision (parent guidance programmes, units for partially-hearing children, integration programmes, etc) for hearing-impaired children was realised. The development of both the peripatetic and audiological services for hearing-impaired children in the UK, and in numerous other countries, can be directly linked to the teachings and endeavours of the Ewings. They were also particularly interested in the development and teaching of speech and their methods were most comprehensively presented in their book *Speech and the Deaf Child* which was published in 1954.

Their speech teaching methods were on the whole similar to those put forward by Sibley Haycock. There were, however, important differences. The Ewings emphasised the use of residual hearing as the prime avenue through which speech could be developed among deaf children and they also described in detail developmental stages leading to speech readiness and articulation readiness. Like Haycock they recommended a synthetic approach to the teaching of speech with special emphasis on the prosodic features of speech. They recognised the importance of reading and writing in speech improvement and they associated speech teaching with the general linguistic development of the child.

They encouraged the audio-visual perception of speech supplemented where necessary by reading and writing. Vibrotactile and kinaesthetic cues and sometimes visual cues in the form of hand analogies were also recommended. They advocated a multisensory approach to the teaching of speech and they believed that the speech intelligibility of deaf children was dependent on three essential conditions – understanding, skill and practice. They were of the opinion that none of these conditions could be acquired by deaf children on their own unless they had the constant help of a sympathetic, knowledgeable and skilful teacher.

In 1964, the Ewings described a new method in the teaching of speech to deaf children which they termed the Simultaneous Listening, Reading and Speaking (LRS) Method. This procedure relies heavily on the use of residual hearing to bring about speech improvement. The teacher reads the material aloud, employing natural prosodic patterns appropriate to the context. As the teacher reads, a pointer is used to simultaneously follow the printed line. The pupil then approximates the teacher's utterance while keeping pace with the movement of the pointer. The Ewings concluded that the LRS Method assisted deaf children in learning to read, hear, comprehend and speak words within a grammatically correct sentence context (Ewing and Ewing, 1964). This was partly verified in a recent experimental study (McMahon and Subtelny, 1981) which reported that the use of the LRS Method brought about significant improvement in the speech intelligibility of deaf students.

By the middle 1960s the era of the Ewings was over. Their influence is still with us but their methods of teaching speech to deaf children are not at present as widely known or practised as they used to be. We have certainly inherited their teaching and writings but we are about to lose their professionalism. Old ideas, clothed in new jargon, are currently put forward as the latest developments in the 'teaching' of speech. Some teachers of the deaf even go as far as to suggest that no 'teaching of speech' is required or that one cannot 'teach' speech as such. They, instead, advocate the use of the residual hearing of the children to its maximum in 'natural' educational environments whereby the teacher does not intervene with regard to the child's speech – the 'natural approach'.

No attempt will be made here to unravel philosophical issues as to what constitutes a 'natural' or an 'unnatural' approach. The danger exists, however, that the term 'natural' and its connotations may be used by certain people to mean the 'right approach', that is their own approach, and any deviation or any other view expressed that is contrary to certain preconceived ideas may be branded as an 'unnatural approach' and therefore an inferior approach.

It needs to be emphasised that very few teachers of the deaf at present would take issue with the beneficial effects of the use of residual hearing – it is well known that speech is best learned through audition. Most of them, however, judging from experience and from indisputable research findings (Ewing, 1967; Duffy, 1967; Erber, 1971) would argue that the use of residual hearing should be supplemented when necessary by the use of visual, tactile and kinaesthetic cues, especially when dealing with very deaf children. The exponents of the 'natural approach' are not very clear on this. For example, it is not clear whether they are advocating a unisensory auditory approach or whether their approach is basically an audio-visual one but with the visual modality not overtly encouraged. It is not clear whether they recommend this approach for all hearing-impaired children irrespective of (a) degree of residual hearing and (b) other audiological and physical complications such as gross interaural frequency disparities, narrow dynamic range of hearing and central speech perceptual disorders.

Also the concept of 'non-intervention' in the teaching of speech as advocated by the exponents of the 'natural approach' is nebulous and, strictly speaking, is incompatible with teacher–pupil interaction. Speech is a learned skill which needs to be taught to most deaf children. As such, the teaching, instructional or developmental process to be followed, implies a degree of intervention by the teacher and there is nothing unnatural about it. Of course, there are gradations of intervention in quantity, quality and manner and it is hoped that the professional involved should be able to adjust his or her degree of intervention according to the abilities and needs of the child.

The exponents of the 'natural approach' have not as yet presented a cohesive account of their principles, objectives and strategies, neither have they the necessary documented evidence to support their case. They seem to believe, however, that all deaf children can acquire intelligible speech solely by their own efforts and through their auditory modality, no matter how damaged it may be. If this is so then the whole approach is tantamount to a denial of the handicapping effects of deafness and it is, to say the least, a very simplistic way of looking at the complexity of the speech problems that can arise as a result of deafness. No further comment on this is necessary. It is too early to judge the relative merits of this approach.

There is no doubt that the most important factor that has influenced the teaching of speech to deaf children in the twentieth century is the use of amplification. We have already mentioned the work of Urbantschitsch from Vienna, Alexander Graham Bell and Goldstein in the USA, Bezold and Kroiss in Germany and Kerr Love in Scotland. Many ingenious mechanical devices were constructed and used to channel sound, with some amplification, into the ears of deaf children. Various versions of the speaking tube were in use such as the Audigene Verrier and the Sexton Ear Tube, the latter being a multiple tube arrangement making it into a group aid (Kerr Love, 1893). Some of these conversation tubes were specially constructed so that the deaf pupils could hear not only their teacher's voice but also their own voices – an early recognition of the significance of the concept of auditory feedback in speech development.

The real breakthrough in hearing aid design came in 1900 when Ferdinand Alt from Vienna produced the first electrical amplification device for the use of the hard of hearing. Since this discovery progress has been moving steadily towards smaller and more versatile amplifying devices which could be worn at all times on the body with comfort and convenience.

Early in this century, carbon electrical hearing aids began to be used. At the beginning of the 1920s 'wireless valves' were used and in a few years time the 'thermionic valve' was invented. These technical developments, coupled with concurrent research into the properties of speech and into the residual hearing of children opened up great possibilities for the construction and use of more powerful hearing aids.

The research in question was mainly carried out in the USA and Great Britain. In 1929, Fletcher working in Bell Telephone Laboratories, New York, published his book *Speech and Hearing* which still remains a classic in this area. In 1936 Ewing, Ewing and Littler carried out an audiometric survey of the capacity to hear among pupils in schools for the deaf in the United Kingdom and their findings substantiated what was already known from Kerr Love's researchers that only a minority of children in schools for the deaf were totally deaf. Similar information came also from USA (Hughson, Ciocco and Palmer, 1939).

In 1933 binaural group hearing aids, designed and produced under the guidance of T. S. Littler and the Ewings at Manchester, were in use in 12 English schools for the deaf. The reports from the schools were unanimous in stating that 'substantial benefit in terms of speech and language development had occurred from regular use of the aids' (Ewing and Ewing, 1938, 1954).

The next great landmark in the development of hearing aids in the United Kingdom was the provision of free hearing aids through the National Health Service. Powerful individual hearing aids were developed and made available towards the end of the 1940s (Medical Research Council, 1947) and since then a plethora of both group and individual aids have been produced: bodyworn aids, ear-level aids, hearing aids in spectacle frames, hearing aids that fit whole in the external auditory meatus, hearing aids that function in an electromagnetic field, radio hearing aids, infra-red aids, binaural aids, hearing aids with multiple microphones and multiple receivers, etc. No attempt will be made here to describe the advantages and disadvantages of all these types of hearing aids. Suffice it to state that in terms of intensity (maximum acoustic outputs obtained varying from 125 dB to 145 dB) and frequency amplification (100 Hz to 8 kHz) and in terms of versatility they can meet the needs of the great majority of hearing-impaired people. These developments enable deaf children to use their residual capacity to hear, thus facilitating, among other things, the acquisition of language and speech skills. There is no doubt that at present hearing aid provision is most adequate. Hearing aids, however, can be effective only when they are consistently and properly used and this is an area that presents a very disturbing picture. In 1969 Martin and Lodge reported that on average 50 per cent of hearing-impaired children in schools for the deaf and in units for partially-hearing children were not making proper use of their individual hearing aids. An even worse situation has been noted recently by the present author (Markides, in preparation *a*).

Another important factor that influenced the teaching of speech to deaf children in the twentieth century was the development and expansion of educational services, especially those for preschool hearing-impaired children. The pioneering experiment in Glasgow with preschool deaf children at the beginning of the century was soon followed by a number of cities in the United Kingdom and by 1938 many schools for the deaf opened their doors to local preschool children. The Education Act of 1944 made this offical when it stated that special educational treatment could begin in nursery schools or classes from the age of 2.

In the middle 1940s programmes in preschool training and parent guidance were established both in the UK and in the USA. The American development was pioneered by Mrs Spencer Tracy who established the John Tracy Clinic at Los Angeles which still provides training for young deaf children and residential and correspondence courses for parents. The British initiative came from the Ewings in Manchester.

Preschool services proved extremely beneficial to both deaf children and their families. Their expansion was very rapid so that at present in the United Kingdom not a single deaf preschool child and his family need go without professional support from a peripatetic teacher of the deaf. The early and consistent use of amplification, coupled with expert supervision and guidance to parents, brought about dramatic changes in the education of hearing-impaired children which in turn influenced the teaching of speech.

The rapid development of the units for partially-hearing and deaf children attached to ordinary schools (from one or two in the late 1940s to nearly five hundred in the early 1980s) and also the extensive integration programmes in mainstream education are, to a large extent, a testimony in favour of early education. This shift in educational provision had a profound effect on the 'traditional' school for deaf or partially-hearing children. The last ten years have shown a steady decrease of numbers of hearing-impaired children attending such schools. This, in conjunction with the recent falling birth rate, may bring about the closure of a considerable number of these schools.

Not only have the numbers of children in most 'traditional' schools for the deaf decreased but also the composition of the children in these schools in terms of additional handicap, degree of hearing loss and linguistic background has changed considerably. It is a fact that the present population of children in most schools for the deaf is on average deafer than it was twenty years ago and also a larger proportion of these children suffer from additional handicap (Warnock, 1979). Also, some schools cater for a larger number of deaf children whose parents are not English speaking.

These changes have affected the teaching of speech both in mainstream education, including units, and in schools for the deaf. In mainstream education the teaching of speech, where practised, does not feature prominently on the timetable. It is true that most of the hearing-impaired children in ordinary schools may not require intensive help with their speech. Some of them, however, do, but in the complex curriculum of the ordinary school their specific needs in speech improvement seem to be forgotten. In most schools for the deaf the teaching of speech still survives but with wide variation from school to school regarding emphasis, method, expertise and expectations.

Overall, educational achievement, especially oral competency among children in many schools for the deaf, is generally low. To a large extent this is most probably due to the potential of the children involved. Other factors, however, such as the school atmosphere, the expectations of the teachers, the calibre of the teachers, the methods of instruction employed or a combination of factors, play a very important part. There is no doubt that many school authorities are examining this situation critically and recently quite a few of them have decided to do something about it and have opted to change their methods of instruction from mainly oral to mainly manual! The use of cued speech, combined methods, Paget Gorman System, British Sign Language, Finger Spelling and more recently 'Total Communication' is widespread. We may be witnessing another flight from oralism.

Other factors, such as increasing parental involvement, state involvement, changes in basic educational philosophy and research have had enormous influence on the teaching of speech in the twentieth century. The first three of these factors will not be considered in detail here. Suffice it to state that associations of parents of deaf children, at present very well organised and active both at local and national level, have traditionally and consistently supported the teaching of speech. This support, however, has recently been undermined, especially by the influence of mass media. Television, for example, has on several occasions seized on the novelty of manual methods of communication and projected them as the most desirable and effective means of educating hearing-impaired children.

The state's role in educational and health services has been steadily increasing. Present developments in these areas could not have been achieved without the support of the state. The development of the health service is of particular importance here mainly because it offered facilities for early diagnosis of deafness and expert medical and surgical intervention when needed. As stated individual hearing aids for both children and adults are provided through the National Health Service and at present a wide variety of types and models are available. Educational philosophy has changed gradually from the nineteenth century concept of 'evangelisation' to the pragmatic realisation in the twentieth century that children require education according to their 'Age, Ability and Aptitude' (Education Act, 1944).

The fourth factor, that is the relevant research and its influence on the teaching of speech will be presented and discussed in the next chapter.

CONCLUDING REMARKS

There is no doubt that there has been progress in the teaching of speech to deaf children: progress from the days when Bonet first suggested his leather tongue to show articulatory positions, and Thomas Braidwood used his spatula type of instrument to manipulate the position of the tongue, to the present with the computerised techniques in speech analysis, synthesis and presentation which baffle most teachers of the deaf! Progress has followed a cyclical growth and has revolved around individual educators – Ramirez de Cárrion, Amman, Heinicke, Braid-wood, Hill, Vatter, Hirsch, Arnold, Alexander Graham Bell, Goldstein, Haycock, the Ewings and so forth.

Is the message that we have to look to leaders in our own time? . . . Surely one of the purposes of a study of history is to learn from our past mistakes for, as George Santayana put it 'Those who do not learn from the past are condemned to relive it.' [Watson, 1980]

CHAPTER TWO

Major studies relating to the speech of deaf children

Within the last fifty years just over one hundred and fifty original papers dealing with the speech of deaf children have been published in professional journals. Most of these papers have reported that deaf children as a group have considerable difficulty in making themselves understood to the general public because of poor speech production skills. No attempt will be made in this chapter to summarise each one of these papers. Only a representative number of them will be presented.

One of the first workers to deal experimentally with the speech of deaf children was Hudgins. In 1934 he compared the speech coordination of 62 deaf and 25 hearing subjects through kymographic tracings as they repeated phrases of nine, seven, five and four syllables containing voiced, unvoiced, nasal and stop consonants. In comparing the speech of the two groups he concluded that the deaf had the following abnormalities:

(*a*) extremely slow and very heavy, laboured speech with inadequate chest pressure;
(*b*) expenditure of an excessive amount of breath for each phrase;
(*c*) substitutions and distortions of vowels and consonants;
(*d*) abnormalities of rhythm;
(*e*) excessive nasal emission;
(*f*) improper functioning of either releasing or arresting consonants;
(*g*) production of inappropriate adventitious syllables.

He recommended that teachers of profoundly deaf children would be helped through understanding the speech coordination of normal children.

Two years later, Hudgins's experiment, with slight modifications, was replicated by Rawlings (1936). He compared the amount of breath consumed by deaf and hearing subjects while breathing quietly and while speaking. He found that the normal speakers used the same amount of air for speaking as for quiet breathing. Among deaf children he found that breath consumption while speaking depended on the degree of hearing loss, the greater the hearing loss the greater the amount of air consumed. In fact his results were similar to those of Hudgins, both experiments supporting each other and suggesting the need for teaching the deaf child a more economical and efficient management of breath control.

Voelker (1935), using the strobophotoscopic system, compared the speech and voice of 28 deaf children when reading ten sentences with the speech and voice of their teachers and a group of normal children. His aim was to determine and measure the effects of the factors of intonation, pitch and duration on the speech of the deaf. He found that, although some of the deaf children showed a tendency towards perseverated pitch patterns, the majority of them were capable of pitch changes as rapid and as extensive as in normal voices. He also stated that the deaf, on average, took almost four times as long and used three times as much phonation in saying a sentence as the normals. In a later study Voelker (1938) reported on the rate of speaking of deaf and normal speakers when reading simple sentences. He found that the mean rate of utterance for normal speakers was 164·4 words per minute. The deaf children showed a wide range of scores with a mean of 69·6 words per minute. He concluded that in the oral education of the deaf the children should be helped to acquire a normal rate of speaking by placing more emphasis on an increased rate of utterance.

A more analytical study of the speech of deaf children was reported in 1936 by Miller-Shaw. He included in his study 10 hearing-impaired adolescents whose intelligence, according to their teachers, was average or above average. He investigated their speech accomplishments following three months intensive speech training during which the 10 children were each given four 40-minute periods of speech teaching each week, using a high fidelity amplifier which made it possible for the children (according to Miller-Shaw) to hear all the speech sounds! He pointed out, however, that although auditory stimulation played the predominant part in the correction technique employed he also supplemented it by using visual, tactile, kinaesthetic and in fact every technique known to him. He pointed out 'as perhaps the most universal characteristic common to every one of the ten subjects' regarding their speech was the frequent reversal of consonants: 'bets' for 'best', 'bakset' for 'basket', 'kate' for 'take', etc. Moreover he stated that none of the subjects pronounced /s/ or /z/ correctly in the three positions (initial, medial and final) – and 7 of the 10 children could not say correctly the voiced velar nasal consonant /ŋ/ as in 'king'. Miller-Shaw was very reluctant to make any generalisations owing to the small sample studied and the relatively short training periods. However, he concluded that the marked improvement in the children's speech intelligibility, spontaneous speech, phrasing and accent amply justified the time and effort expended on training.

Five years afterwards the implications of Miller-Shaw's study regarding methodologies of teaching speech to deaf children were taken up by Hughson, Ciocco, Whitting and Lawrence (1941). Their sample of 366 deaf children was divided into two groups, one of which had been taught by the 'auricular' method, the other by the 'oral' method. The test administered to the children consisted of 26 words known to young deaf children. This list of words, according to the authors, included all vowels and consonants with the latter being tested in initial and final positions as far as was possible. The children were asked to read these words and their speech was recorded on 12-inch cellulose acetate discs. The same test was also administered to a group of hearing children whose speech was recorded for comparative purposes. The following speech characteristics were studied: articulation, explosiveness and audibility of the first and final consonants, holding or duration of vowels, syllable continuity and expression. Their final evaluation indicated that children from 'auricular' classes were superior in speech intelligibility when compared with children taught by 'oral' methods. However, Dale (1958) considered their findings to be invalid on the grounds of lack of information regarding the sampling technique used to select the two groups of children and the omission of any information on the residual capacity of the children to hear. It is also pointed out that the above writers failed to give any precise definition of their 'auricular' and 'oral' methods of teaching speech.

There is no doubt that the most intensive study of the intelligibility of the speech of deaf children was conducted by Hudgins and Numbers (1942). They recorded speech samples of 192 deaf pupils from ages 8 to 20 with hearing losses ranging from a slight impairment to profound deafness. The pupils were drawn from two oral schools for the deaf. The test materials employed consisted of 1200 unrelated simple sentences which were grouped in tens. Each pupil was provided with one group of sentences which he read after practice, his speech being recorded phonographically on either aluminium or acetate discs. The records were then played to groups of listeners who had some experience with the speech of the deaf. Each recorded sentence was replayed three times and the auditors were required to write on paper what they thought the child had said. The speech intelligibility scores were determined as follows: ten points were given for sentences written correctly, no points being awarded for partially correct interpretations. Moreover the records were also analysed to determine the frequency and type of both rhythmic and articulatory errors committed and their relationship to intelligibility.

The sentences in the test were divided into three groups according to rhythm: those spoken with normal rhythm (approximately 45%), those spoken with abnormal rhythm (approximately 35%) and those spoken without rhythm (approximately 20%). The chief characteristics of the sentences spoken with abnormal rhythm were the unusual groupings of the words and syllables in the sentence and the atypical stress patterns affecting both place and degree. The non-rhythmical sentences exhibited monotonous stress patterns with all vowel-like sounds in the sentence equally affected. They found a high correlation between rhythmic errors and poor intelligibility. Sentences spoken with normal rhythm were understood four times as often as those sentences spoken with incorrect rhythm.

Hudgins and Numbers also analysed all rhythmic sentence categories according to degree of hearing loss and age. They found an increase in the number of sentences spoken with normal rhythm with increasing amount of residual hearing and a decrease in the number of sentences spoken non-rhythmically with increasing age.

The articulatory errors of the deaf children were assigned into two major errors: errors involving vowels and errors involving consonants. The vowel errors revealed vowel substitution, non-functioning of the diphthong (splitting the diphthong into two distinct vowels or omitting one member of the diphthong usually the final one), nasalisation of vowels, neutralisation and diphthongisation of simple vowels. Among other consonant errors the deaf children failed to distinguish between surd and sonant consonants, they substituted consonants, they produced consonants with excessive nasality, they misarticulated compound consonants and they failed to produce releasing and arresting consonants adequately.

The writers also analysed all the articulatory errors according to degree of hearing loss and age. In the first instance they found that as hearing loss increased a greater number of errors occurred. In detail they stated that consonant substitutions and errors involving compound and arresting consonants were more numerous among the hard of hearing than among the profoundly deaf pupils. In the second instance they found that consonant errors increased with age whilst vowel errors showed very little change. They argued that, since frequency of articulatory errors and speech intelligibility scores were negatively correlated, the speech of the older pupils was less intelligible than that of the younger children. However, they made the above statement with some reservation mainly because the degree of hearing loss among the pupils of individual age groups was not the same. Nevertheless, their findings tend to agree with Haycock's statement (1933) that 'It is commonly observed that the speech of deaf-born pupils becomes less intelligible as they advance from the lower to the higher classes in school.'

The general conclusion was that speech intelligibility depended considerably on the proper articulation of phonemes and on the rhythmic pattern of the sentence. They indicated that the speech errors of the deaf children may have been due to the analytical method of teaching speech used in the schools concerned. They recommended the use of syllables rather than isolated phonemes in the teaching of speech.

Following this study, Hudgins became very interested in the breathing habits of deaf children and in 1946 he reported on the relationship between speech breathing and speech intelligibility among deaf pupils. In this pioneer study he referred to five anomalous breathing habits characterising the speech of deaf talkers:

(a) short irregular breath groups often only one or two words in length with breath pauses interrupting the speech flow at improper points;

(b) excessive expenditure of breath on single syllables resulting in breathy speech;

(c) false grouping of syllables resulting in the breaking up of natural groups and misplacement of accents;

(d) a slow methodical utterance resulting in a complete lack of groupings; and

(e) a lack of proper coordination between breathing muscles and articulatory organs.

He found a marked reduction in speech intelligibility due to poor breathing habits thus emphasising the importance of good and appropriate respiratory controls.

A study conducted by Sheridan regarding the child's hearing for speech was published in book form in 1948. A section of this study dealt with the speech of 100 hearing-impaired children who were singled out after an audiometric survey of the school populations of Salford, Lancashire. Sheridan found that 57 of these children had speech defects. She examined their speech by engaging each child in conversation or having each child describe colourful pictures. When a sound was determined defective she gave the child sentences to read involving that sound. She made no attempt to standardise her examination procedure and it is obvious that the above method of examining the speech of the children was a very personal one. She reported that the commonest fault in the speech of the hearing-impaired children was either a defective /s/ or its omission, particularly at the end and in the middle of words. She also found defects of /r/ very common but as a degeneration of the sound rather than as a substitution. She found vowel substitution rare. In conclusion she stated that the greater the degree of deafness the more distorted was the speech of these children. She found girls superior to boys in speech skills.

In 1953 Clark studied two similar groups of profoundly deaf children ($n = 23$ in each group). The children in one group received two 45-minute periods of auditory training each week for a period of one school year. He concluded that at the end of the year the children who received his training showed statistically significant improvements in language development, speech perception, intelligibility, rhythm and rate of speaking. Regarding speech intelligibility he asserted that consonants were more important for intelligibility than vowels and that the total number of articulation errors gave the best predicted value of intelligibility.

Sanders's investigation (1961) concerning the progress made since entry to school by a group of 50 deaf children who received preschool training and early use of an individual hearing aid, contained information on the speech intelligibility and voice production of 41 of these children. He assessed their speech intelligibility during the testing period whilst they were describing a set of pictures. Assessment was done on a six-point scale. His results showed little difficulty in understanding the speech of the majority of the children. In comparing the ratings of the speech intelligibility of the children with their hearing loss he found a definite relationship, i.e. the speech of the children with a slight hearing impairment was better than the speech of children with more severe hearing impairment. At the time of rating intelligibility he also made a subjective evaluation of the degree of impairment of each child's voice. This was done on the following four-point scale:

(a) normal voice,
(b) voice slightly affected,
(c) voice moderately affected,
(d) voice severely affected.

He found a definite relationship between the severity of the hearing loss and the degree of impairment of voice. He stated that children with hearing losses of less than 75 dB did not exhibit more than a slight impairment of voice quality whilst children with losses of 75 dB or over showed definite defects in voice quality. It is only fair to state, however, that Sanders himself was rather sceptical about the validity of his findings regarding this aspect.

The main aim of Johnson's study (1962) was to obtain information with regard to the educational attainments and social adjustment of hearing-impaired children. Out of the 66 children studied, he reported that 54 had speech defects. He asserted that type of hearing impairment rather than degree of hearing loss was the main factor affecting speech intelligibility. He stated that children suffering from 'perceptive' deafness nearly always develop defective speech. The results of his study led him to believe that hearing-impaired children develop considerably greater fluency of speech in a normal school environment where they have the opportunity of mixing with hearing children rather than in a special school where this opportunity is lacking.

Carlin (1964) compared the speech improvement of two groups of partially-hearing children. One of the groups was provided with special help for a period of one year whilst the other group did not receive special help. His main conclusions were that the children who received special help made a significant 63 per cent reduction in their consonant articulation errors whilst the children who did not receive such help made only a 27 per cent improvement. He also stated that the consonant articulation errors of some of the children who did not receive special help actually increased in the course of a year. In analysing the consonant errors of the children he found that the most frequently misarticulated consonants were /s/, /θ/, /z/ and /ð/. He was of the opinion that the pronunciation of the first three of the above consonants could be improved considerably with special teaching but not without it. He stated that the most frequent type of error was the substitution of one phoneme for another and he noticed that omissions of consonants in the initial and medial positions were rare whilst omissions in the final position were relatively common.

John and Howarth (1965) studied the effects of time distortions on the intelligibility of speech of deaf children. Recognising that many of the errors in the speech of such children may be described as those of abnormal time relationships, an attempt was made to improve the speech intelligibility of a group of 29 severely deaf children by focusing teaching on this aspect of their speech. The children were selected at random from three schools. Due to lack of information only two factors that might have affected the children's speech intelligibility were examined statistically, namely hearing loss and age. Twenty-nine short spontaneous sentences, one from each child, were recorded on tape both initially, before any teaching was carried out, and finally after three or four minutes teaching designed to improve only the time aspect of the speech. The speech intelligibility of the children was judged by 20 lay university students who were required to write down as much as they could of the initial and final versions of the children's recorded speech. The judges' interpretations were scored in two ways, first on the number of words understood correctly and secondly on the recognition of the completed syntactic pattern of the children's speech. Using the first method of scoring an improvement in intelligibility of 56 per cent between the initial and final versions was found. When scoring by the second method the improvement noted rose to 203 per cent. There was no statistical difference in improvement on the basis of either hearing loss or age. They concluded by stating that teaching that stressed the temporal aspects of speech, relying heavily on the auditory feedback of speech patterns as wholes, was a quick and effective means of improving speech intelligibility in deaf children. Note, however, that Boothroyd, Nickerson and Stevens (1974) have found that methodologies of teaching speech to deaf children which rely solely on the rhythmic aspects of speech have very little to recommend them. In view of this it would be desirable (a) to replicate John and Howarth's experiment in order to ascertain the test–retest reliability of results obtained; (b) to expand the experiment to deal with groups of children having varying degrees of speech intelligibility;* (c) to ascertain whether similar, or even better results, cannot be obtained by other methods of direct speech teaching; and (d) to investigate the long-term effects of the teaching method suggested – the improvements reported related only to a single very short speech teaching session.

Markides' (1967) study on the speech of hearing-impaired children contained information on the articulatory errors and overall speech intelligibility of 58 junior deaf children (hearing loss in the better ear, averaged across the frequencies 250–4000 Hz, in excess of 80 dB HL) and 27 partially-hearing children (averaged hearing loss less than 80 dB HL). The results of this study will be presented in detail later on. It is of interest to note here, however, that the deaf children misarticulated 56 per cent of the vowels and diphthongs and 72 per cent of the consonants included in the articulation test. Inexperienced listeners were able to understand correctly only 19 per cent of the words spoken by the deaf children.

In 1967 Nober used the Templin–Darley Test of Articulation with a view to studying the articulatory error patterns of deaf children. His investigation included 46 hearing-impaired children varying in age from 3 to 15 years. He found that when the hearing loss exceeded 80 dB HL for the main speech frequencies, none of the children achieved the minimum testable age level norms of 3 years. In fact none of the children with hearing losses of 60–80 dB HL scored higher than the 4-year age level. He found articulation proficiency increasing with age but surprisingly he reported a weak relationship between articulatory skill and degree of hearing loss. Nober also reported the following four important findings:

(a) There was high correlation between correct articulation and degree of consonant visibility.
(b) Diphthongs were associated with the highest frequency of correct production, followed by stops, nasals and fricatives.
(c) Consonant blends were rarely produced correctly,
(d) Vowels and diphthongs were much more easier articulated than consonants.

Finally, in a recent study Ling and Milne (1979) provided a very optimistic picture regarding the speech potential of hearing-impaired children. They evaluated the speech of 7 profoundly hearing-impaired children (average HL in the better ear ranging from 85 dB to 105 dB) who were trained from early infancy in a special project. The goals of their study were threefold: first, to evaluate the speech attainments of the 7

---

* It is important to remember that the degree of improvement depends upon the original percentage score for speech intelligibility. If this is low then an elevation of 50 per cent or even 200 per cent may not be as dramatic as it sounds.

children; second, to determine the extent to which their spoken language sounded similar to that of their normally hearing peers of the same age and sex; and finally, to examine certain suprasegmental features of speech relating to judgements of normality. The peer comparison revealed that the speech intelligibility of the hearing-impaired children was not significantly poorer than that of their normally hearing counterparts. Ling and Milne contended that levels of intelligibility ranging between 56 and 98 per cent could be attained, and that with adequate, well planned training the deviant characteristics of deaf children's speech could be overcome and fluent intelligible speech could be attained by most hearing-impaired children. They found that intonation, voice pitch, stress, rhythm and vowel production were correlated with speech intelligibility but surprisingly quality was not. They stated that speech faults such as poor voice quality, prolongation, neutralisation or diphthongisation of vowels, intrusive voicing, nasalisation and voiced–voiceless errors, all very common errors associated with the speech of hearing-impaired children, were not evident in the samples of speech of the children included in their study. Ling (1976) was of the opinion that these errors were not so much related to deafness, as some previous studies suggested, but to the type of treatment the children received, usually one of benign neglect or inappropriate therapy practices.

SUMMARY

The researches so far outlined are of particular importance because (a) they have documented the errors involved in the speech of deaf children, (b) they have provided information on the overall speech intelligibility of deaf children, (c) they have highlighted the major factors affecting speech intelligibility, and (d) they have developed various methods and procedures for the assessment of the different parameters of the speech of deaf children.

Broadly speaking the errors noted can be conveniently grouped under two major categories: errors involving the articulatory aspects of speech, and errors of prosody. Of course, such a classification is an oversimplification since acoustically these two categories interpenetrate. Nevertheless the labels provide a useful framework within which the different errors can be presented and discussed. This will be done in the next two chapters.

With regard to overall speech intelligibility the picture presented in these studies is rather gloomy. This is a very important aspect of the speech of deaf children and deserves a more thorough treatment. In view of this the intelligibility of the speech of deaf children, followed by the major factors that have been found to affect it, such as degree of hearing loss, use of residual hearing, schooling, linguistic development and speech teaching will be presented and discussed in more detail in Chapter 5.

The methods and procedures involved in the assessment of the different parameters of the speech of deaf children are of particular importance and they will be treated in Chapter 6.

PART II

Speech attainments and speech disorders

JABBERWOCKY

'Twas brillig, and the slithy toves
    Did gyre and gimble in the wabe:
All mimsy were the borogoves,
    And the mome raths outgrabe.

'Beware the Jabberwock, my son!
    The jaws that bite, the claws that catch!
Beware the Jujub bird, and shun
    The frumious Bandersnatch!'

He took his vorpal sword in hand:
    Long time the manxome foe he sought—
So rested he by the Tumtum tree,
    And stood awhile in thought.

And, as in uffish thought he stood,
    The Jabberwock, with eyes of flame,
Came whiffling through the tulgey wood,
    And burbled as it came!

One, two! One, two! And through and through
    The vorpal blade went snicker-snack!
He left it dead, and with its head
    He went galumphing back.

'And hast thou slain the Jabberwock?
    Come to my arms, my beamish boy!
O frabjous day! Callooh! Callay!'
    He chortled in his joy.

'Twas brillig, and the slithy toves
    Did gyre and gimble in the wabe:
All mimsy were the borogoves,
    And the mome raths outgrabe.

'It seems very pretty,' she said when she had finished it, 'but it's *rather* hard to understand! Somehow it seems to fill my head with ideas—only I don't exactly know what they are! However, *somebody* killed *something*: that's clear, at any rate—'

Lewis Carroll: *Through the Looking-Glass*

CHAPTER THREE

Articulatory features

In the preceding chapter some general observations were made concerning the articulatory errors in the speech of deaf children. In the present chapter, more specific data pertaining to these articulatory errors will be presented and discussed.

The most comprehensive study of the speech of deaf children was carried out by Hudgins and Numbers in 1942. A large section of the study dealt with the articulatory skills of the children but this will not be presented here mainly because the research work in question was carried out forty years ago at a time when deaf children were not enjoying the benefits of modern hearing aids. In view of this the results are largely out of date and therefore it would be more appropriate to concentrate on recent studies. This chapter will be primarily concerned with the articulatory results reported in two studies completed by the present author in 1967 and in 1980 (Markides, 1967, 1980*b*).

THE 1967 STUDY

This study has already been mentioned in the previous chapter. It dealt with the speech of 58 deaf and 27 partially-hearing children. The deaf children on average were 8 years 5 months old (range 7 years to 10 years) and the partially-hearing averaged 8 years 4 months with a similar age range.

The mean hearing loss of the deaf children was nearly 95 dB (averaged across the frequencies 250 Hz to 4000 Hz in the better ear) with a range of 70 dB to 115 dB. The partially-hearing children on average showed a hearing loss of 57 dB (range 40 dB to 75 dB). The great majority of these children (95% of the deaf and 50% of the partially-hearing) were either born deaf or acquired their hearing loss during the first year of life.

The articulation test used (see Table 3.1) was constructed by the writer

TABLE 3.1   Articulation test

| | Phonemes tested | | |
Word	initially (I)	medially (M)	finally (F)
1 pig	p	ɪ	g
2 ship	ʃ		p
3 boy	b		ɔɪ
4 ball		ɔ	l
5 bath		ɑ	θ
6 book		ʊ	k
7 cat	k	æ	t
8 dog	d	ɒ	
9 red	r	ɛ	d
10 gun	g	ʌ	n
11 chair	tʃ		ɛə
12 watch	w		tʃ
13 moon	m	u	
14 farm	f		m
15 knife	n	aɪ	f
16 swing			ŋ
17 fish			ʃ
18 house	h	aʊ	s
19 sun	s		
20 girl		ɜ	
21 five			v
22 ten	t		
23 keys		i	z
24 zoo	z		

as none was available and it was based on the above 24 monosyllabic words which were represented pictorially on separate cards 6 cm × 8 cm (Appendix 1). The words included in the articulation test were specially chosen to be within the vocabulary of the children and to test a representative number of vowels, diphthongs and consonants in the English language. The responses of the children to the articulation test were recorded on magnetic tape and later on transcribed in phonetic script.

The vowel and diphthong errors of the children were assigned to five categories.

1 *Vowel substitution*: Substitution of one vowel for another as of /ɒ/ for /ɪ/ in the pronunciation of [ʃɒp] for [ʃɪp] or of /ʌ/ for /ɒ/ in [dʌg] for [dɒg].
2 *Vowel neutralisation*: This category included all errors where the neutral vowel /ə/ was substituted for another vowel. For example, /ə/

for /ɪ/ in the pronunciation of [pəg] for [pɪg] or of /ə/ for /ɛ/ in [rəd] for [rɛd].

3 *Vowel prolongation*: The errors included in this category were the ones where vowels were excessively prolonged. For example, /uː/ for /u/ as in the pronunciation of [muːn] for [mun] or of /ɔː/ for /ɔ/ in [bɔːl] for [bɔl].

4 *Vowel diphthongisation*: This category included all errors where vowels were produced as diphthongs. For example, /ɔɪ/ for /ɒ/ in the pronunciation of [dɔɪg] [dɒg] or of /oʊ/ for /ɔ/ in [boʊl] for [bɔl].

5 *Diphthong errors*: These were mainly of three kinds:

(a) Usually the first component of the glide was excessively prolonged thus resulting in the diphthong being heard as two distinct vowels. For example, /ɔːːɪ/ for /ɔɪ/ in the pronunciation of [bɔːːɪ] for [bɔɪ] and /aːːʊ/ for /aʊ/ in [háːːʊs] for [háʊs].

(b) One of the components of the diphthong, usually the final one, was dropped, the remaining one being excessively prolonged as of /ɔː/ for /ɔɪ/ in the pronunciation of [bɔː] for [bɔɪ] or of /ɛː/ for /ɛə/ in [tʃɛː] for [tʃɛə].

(c) The diphthong was heard as the neutral vowel /ə/. For example, /ə/ for /aɪ/ in the pronunciation of [nəf] for [naɪf] or of /ə/ for /ɔɪ/ in [bə] for [bɔɪ].

The consonant errors of the children were assigned to three categories:

1 *Omission*: The failure to produce a sound in the position in which it should occur and the failure to insert any other sound in its place. For example, an omission of final /t/ is noted in the pronunciation of [kæ] for [kæt].

2 *Substitution*: The use of one speech sound in place of another as of /v/ for /f/ in the pronunciation of [naɪv] for [naɪf], or of /t/ for /b/ in [tɔl] for [bɔl].

3 *Distortion*: The faulty production of a speech sound, although the sound produced is recognised as being an example of the desired phoneme. For example, a whistled or lateral /s/ may be considered a distortion of the /s/ sound.

VOWEL AND DIPHTHONG ERRORS

The deaf children (*N* = 58) made 482 vowel and diphthong errors, an average of 8·32 errors per child. The partially-hearing children (*N* = 27) made 35 vowel and diphthong errors, an average of 1·29 errors per child. In the first instance the errors amounted to nearly 56 per cent of all vowels and diphthongs attempted whilst in the second instance the errors amounted to approximately 9 per cent. Figure 3.1 shows the distribution of vowel and diphthong errors according to individual error categories.

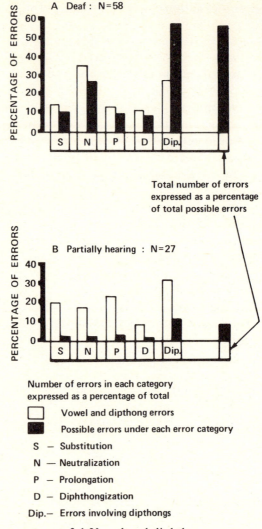

Total number of errors
expressed as a percentage
of total possible errors

Number of errors in each category
expressed as a percentage of total

☐   Vowel and dipthong errors

■   Possible errors under each error category

S — Substitution

N — Neutralization

P — Prolongation

D — Diphthongization

Dip.— Errors involving dipthongs

FIGURE 3.1 Vowel and diphthong errors

It can be noted that category 2 (vowel neutralisation) included by far the greatest number (just over 35%) of errors made by the deaf children. Errors involving diphthongs follow this closely, accounting for 27 per cent of their total errors. The remaining three categories each contained similar percentages of the total errors made by the deaf children, i.e. 11 to 13 per cent.

For the partially-hearing children, errors involving diphthongs were the most numerous (31% of their errors). These were followed by errors involving vowel prolongation, vowel substitution and vowel neutralisation with each one accounting for roughly the same percentage of the total number of errors made by the partially-hearing children, i.e. 17 to 22 per cent.

When the errors in each category were expressed as percentages of total possible errors it was found that both the deaf and the partially-hearing children had more difficulty with the pronunciation of diphthongs. The actual vowel and diphthong errors made by the children are shown in Table 3.2.

Vowel substitution

Amongst the deaf children the most substitutions were made for the short vowel /ɪ/ as in 'pig' (14 times), followed by the vowels /ɑ/ as in 'bath' (10 times), and the vowels /ʌ/ as in 'gun' and /ɜ/ in 'girl' (8 times each). The substitutions were not limited to adjacent vowels or to vowels of a similar formation, as in /i/ for /ɪ/. For example, the back vowel /ɔ/ as in 'ball' was substituted for the high front long vowel /i/ in 3 instances, and for the high front short vowel /ɪ/ in 4 instances. The front vowel /ɛ/ was substituted for the back vowel /ʊ/ in 2 instances, and for /u/ in 3.

The partially-hearing children made 7 substitution errors. /ɔ/ was substituted once for /i/ and once for /æ/, /i/ was substituted twice for /ɪ/, /ʊ/ was substituted twice for /ɑ/ and /ɒ/ was substituted once for /ʊ/.

Vowel neutralisation

In this category the most frequently neutralised phonemes amongst the deaf children were the vowels /æ/ as in 'cat' (29 times), and /ɛ/ as in 'red' (26 times). The partially-hearing children neutralised the vowels /ɪ/, /ɛ/ and /ʊ/ once each.

Vowel prolongation

Prolongations amongst the deaf and partially-hearing children occurred mainly with the back vowels /ɒ/, /ɔ/, /u/ and /ʊ/ which accounted for nearly 90 per cent of all errors included in this category. For example, 17 children (16 deaf and 1 partially-hearing) produced the short vowel /ɒ/ as /ɔː/; 14 children (11 deaf and 3 partially-hearing) prolonged excessively the vowel /ɔ/ which was heard as /ɔː/; 11 children (8 deaf and 3 partially-hearing) prolonged excessively the vowel /u/ which was heard as /uː/ and 9 deaf children produced the short vowel /ʊ/ as /uː/.

Vowel diphthongisation

Diphthongisation of vowels was the least common mistake made by both deaf and partially-hearing children. Amongst the deaf children diphthongisation affected all vowels, the most commonly diphthongised being /ɒ/ as in 'dog' (8 times) and /i/ as in 'keys' (7 times); /ɒ/ was heard 5

TABLE 3.2 Vowel and diphthong errors made by deaf (N = 58) and partially-hearing children (N = 27)

	Vowels											Diphthongs			
	i	ɪ	ɛ	æ	ɑ	ʌ	ɜ	ɒ	ɔ	ʊ	u	aɪ	aʊ	ɔɪ	ɛə
Number of errors made by the deaf	28	36	36	37	24	40	31	38	27	28	26	38	22	30	41
Number of errors made by the partially-hearing	1	4	1	1	2	3	1	2	3	2	4	3	1	2	5
Errors made by the deaf	14/ə 4/iː 4/ɪə 3/ɪʊ 2/ɔ 1/ʊ	14/ə 6/i 5/iː 4/ɛ 4/ɔ 3/ɪə	25/ə 3/ɪ 3/ɛə 2/ɪə 2/ɛː 1/oʊ	29/ə 3/aɪ 2/ɛə 2/ʊ 1/ɔ	10/ə 2/ɑː 4/ʊ 4/ɔ 2/ʊə 2/ɛə	25/ə 4/æ 2/u 2/ʊ 2/ʌ 2/ɛə 3/ɔə	18/ə 4/ʊ 2/i 2/ɔ 1/ɪː 2/ɛə 2/ɪə	16/ɔː 10/ə 2/ɔ 2/ɑ 5/ɔɪ 3/oʊ	11/ɔː 6/ə 2/ʊ 2/u 3/ɔə 3/ɔɪ	10/ə 9/uː 2/ɒ 2/ɛ 1/u 2/ʊə 2/əə	8/ə 8/uː 3/ɔ 3/ɛ 3/ʊ 1/ʊə	22/ə 10/aːɪ 1/iː 2/aːɪ 3/aːɪ	12/ə 4/aːɪ 4/uː 2/aːʊ	4/ə 11/ɔːɪ 3/ɔːɪ 11/ɔː 1/iː	13/ə 20/ɛː 8/ɛːə
Errors made by the partially-hearing	1/ɔ	2/i 1/ə 1/ɪə	1/ə	1/ɔ	2/ʊ	3/ə	1/ɜː	1/ɒː 1/oʊ	3/ɔː	1/ɒ 1/ə	3/uː 1/ɪʊ	2/ə 1/aː	1/ə	2/ɔːɪ	3/ɜː 1/ɛɜ 1/ə

times as /ɔɪ/ and 3 times as /oʊ/; /i/ was heard 4 times as /ɪə/ and 3 times as /ɪʊ/.

Amongst the partially-hearing children there were 3 diphthongisations associated with the vowels /ɪ/, /ɒ/ and /u/. Vowel /ɪ/ was heard as /ɪə/, /ɒ/ as /oʊ/ and /u/ as /ɪʊ/.

Errors involving diphthongs

The deaf children misarticulated over 56 per cent of all diphthongs attempted. The partially-hearing children misarticulated just over 10 per cent of all diphthongs they attempted.

Both the deaf and the partially-hearing children had most difficulty with the diphthongs /ɛə/ and /aɪ/. Their commonest mistake was to substitute the neutral vowel /ə/ for the diphthong. Thus /aɪ/ as in 'knife' was heard as /ə/, [nəf], and /ɔɪ/ as in 'boy' was heard as /ə/, [bə].

The next most common mistake was to drop the second component of the diphthong, at the same time prolonging its first component. For example, /aɪ/ as in 'knife' was heard as /aː/, [naːf] with or without the final /f/.

Finally, the excessive prolongation, usually of the first component of the glide, resulting in the diphthong being heard as two distinct vowels, constituted the least common diphthong mistake. For example, the diphthong /ɔɪ/ as in 'boy' was heard as /ɔːɪ/ [bɔːɪ] or /ɛə/ as in 'chair' was heard as /ɛːə/ [tʃɛːə].

CONSONANT ERRORS

The deaf children made 1336 consonant errors, nearly 72 per cent of all consonants attempted, and an average of 23·01 errors per child. Of these errors, 622, an average of 10·72 errors per child, were associated with initial consonants, whilst the remaining 714, an average of 12·31 errors per child, were associated with final consonants.

The partially-hearing children made 228 consonant errors, a little over 26 per cent of all consonants attempted and an average of 8·44 errors per child. A total of 89 of their errors, an average of 3·29 errors per child, were associated with initial consonants, whilst the remaining 139, an average of 5·13 errors per child, were associated with final consonants. This information for both deaf and partially-hearing children is shown in Figures 3.2 to 3.4.

It can be noted then that the partially-hearing children made comparatively fewer consonant errors than the deaf children and that for both the deaf and the partially-hearing children errors involving the final consonants were more numerous than errors involving the initial consonants.

When the consonant errors were divided into omissions, substitutions

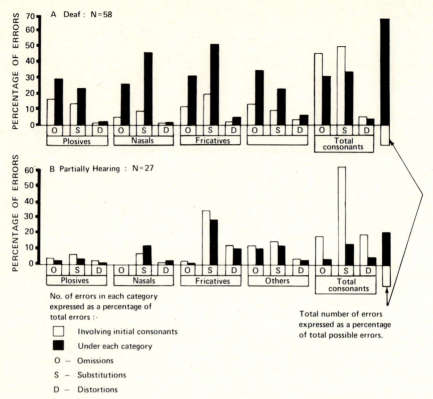

FIGURE 3.2 Consonant errors according to manner of production (initial position)

and distortions it was found that just over 63 per cent of all the deaf children's consonant errors were omissions, nearly 30 per cent were substitutions and the remaining 7 per cent were distortions. For the partially-hearing children substitution errors were the most numerous (45·61%), followed by omission errors (39·91%) and distortions (14·47% of all their consonant errors).

Further analysis into those errors affecting the initial consonants and into those affecting the final consonants showed some interesting results. For example, omissions of final consonants were much more numerous than omissions of initial consonants for both the deaf and the partially-hearing children. Consonant substitutions showed the opposite picture, substitution errors being more numerous with the initial consonants than with the final consonants for both the deaf and the partially-hearing children.

The consonants in the test material were divided according to their manner of production into four groups:

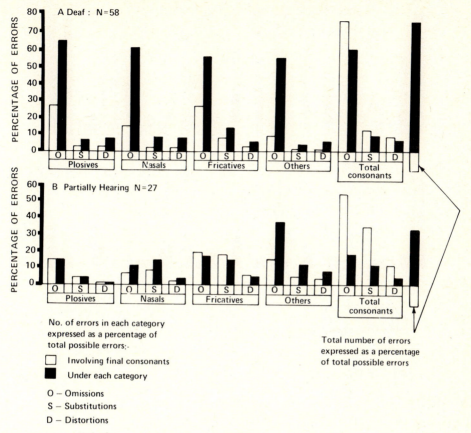

FIGURE 3.3 Consonant errors according to manner of production (final position)

(a) plosives   /p, b, t, d, k, g/
(b) nasals   /m, n, ŋ/
(c) fricatives /f, v, θ, s, z, ʃ/
(d) others   /tʃ, l, r, w, h/

The actual consonant errors made by the children are shown in Tables 3.3 and 3.4.

Plosive consonants

If a complete obstruction is set up in the oral chambers so that no breath can escape, then additional pressure is built up against this closure; and finally if this closure is suddenly broken and the breath released, there is created one of a group of consonants known as plosives. A further essential aspect of this complete closure is that the velum is pressed firmly against the back wall of the oral pharynx, so that none of the breath escapes through the nasal passages. Like most other consonants, these

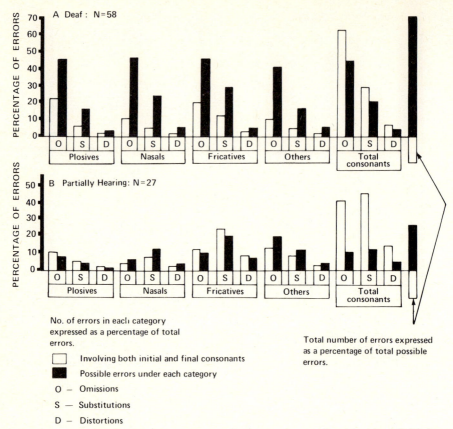

No. of errors in each category
expressed as a percentage of total
errors.

☐   Involving both initial and final consonants

■   Possible errors under each category

O — Omissions

S — Substitutions

D — Distortions

Total number of errors expressed
as a percentage of total possible
errors.

FIGURE 3.4 Consonant errors according to manner of production (initial
and final positions)

plosives may be accompanied by vibration of the vocal folds, in which
case these are 'voiced' plosives. When there is no such vibration the
plosive is said to be 'unvoiced'.

The deaf children made 425 plosive consonant errors. Of these, 296
were omissions, 105 were substitutions and 24 distortions. The partially-
hearing children made 39 plosive errors: 24 omissions, 12 substitutions
and 3 distortions. The most frequently omitted plosive consonants
amongst the deaf children were /g/ in 76 instances (26 times initially and
50 times finally), /d/ in 68 instances (23 times initially, 45 times finally),
and /k/ in 63 instances (25 times initially, 38 times finally). Amongst the
partially-hearing children the most frequently omitted plosive consonants were /d/ in 7 instances when tested finally, /g/ in 6 instances (2
initially and 4 finally) and final /t/ in 5 instances.

Plosive consonants were mainly substituted for plosives. There was a
tendency for the unvoiced plosive consonants to be substituted for their
voiced cognates. For example, among the deaf children, /p/ was

TABLE 3.3 Consonant errors made by the deaf children (N = 58)

Consonants	Plosives						Nasals			Fricatives							Others			
	p	b	t	d	k	g	m	n	ŋ	f	v	θ	s	z	ʃ	tʃ	l	r	w	h
Number of errors in initial position	15	20	27	34	45	49	45	42	57	37	N.T.	N.T.	58	47	58	42	N.T.	31	31	38
Number of errors in final position	37	N.T.	44	55	46	53	37	43	57	36	39	37	52	55	46	46	30	N.T.	N.T.	38
Errors in initial position	8/o/ 3/t/ 2/m/ 1/d/ 1/f/	7/o/ 7/p/ 2/t/ 1/n/ 1/mp/ 2/x/	14/o/ 4/k/ 2/h/ 2/tʃ/ 1/j/ 1/ʒ/ 1/p/ 1/d/ 1/x/	23/o/ 3/t/ 3/j/ 2/k/ 1/z/ 1/h/ 1/p/	25/o/ 9/t/ 6/j/ 4/h/ 1/x/	26/o/ 8/t/ 5/k/ 3/p/ 3/h/ 4/j/	11/o/ 22/p/ 5/t/ 3/b/ 3/f/ 1/x/	20/o/ 11/t/ 4/p/ 2/j/ 2/l/ 1/k/ 1/f/ 1/h/		10/o/ 14/p/ 9/t/ 4/m/	N.T.	N.T.	17/o/ 26/t/ 5/st/ 2/ʃ/ 1/tʃ/ 1/f/ 1/g/ 1/k/ 4/x/	22/o/ 6/n/ 5/ʒ/ 4/t/ 3/k/ 2/dʒ/ 1/h/ 1/ʃ/ 3/x/	20/o/ 22/t/ 3/dʒ/ 3/j/ 3/p/ 3/ʒ/ 1/f/ 3/x/	19/o/ 5/t/ 2/ʃ/ 1/j/ 1/dʒ/ 1/ʒ/ 13/x/	N.T.	11/o/ 6/t/ 4/v/ 3/n/ 3/f/ 2/p/ 2/d/	15/o/ 5/p/ 4/ʊ/ 3/t/ 2/f/ 1/m/ 1/n/	35/o/ 3/t/
Errors in final position	20/o/ 1/t/ 16/x/	N.T.	40/o/ 1/h/ 1/n/ 2/x/	45/o/ 7/t/ 2/k/ 1/s/	38/o/ 5/t/ 1/tʃ/ 2/x/	50/o/ 2/h/ 1/n/	20/o/ 2/t/ 1/p/ 1/n/ 13/x/	35/o/ 4/t/ 1/ʃ/ 1/k/ 2/x/	52/o/ 4/n/ 1/p/	25/o/ 5/ʊ/ 2/p/ 1/p/ 4/x/	27/o/ 2/t/ 2/p/ 2/b/ 2/m/ 1/n/ 3/x/	21/o/ 7/t/ 1/m/ 8/x/	40/o/ 3/p/ 2/f/ 2/t/ 1/m/ 1/ʃ/ 3/x/	47/o/ 5/ʃ/ 2/s/ 1/ʒ/	36/o/ 2/f/ 2/t/ 1/p/ 1/tʃ/ 1/ʒ/ 3/x/	34/o/ 5/ʃ/ 7/x/	30/o/			

/o/ = omissions; / / = substitutions with the sounds substituted; /x/ = distortions. N.T. = not tested.

TABLE 3.4 Consonant errors made by the partially-hearing children ($N = 27$)

Consonants	Plosives						Nasals			Fricatives							Others			
	p	b	t	d	k	g	m	n	ŋ	f	v	θ	s	z	ʃ	tʃ	l	r	w	h
Number of errors in initial position	3	N.T.	5	1	3	8	5	2		5	N.T.	N.T.	12	14	12	9	N.T.	8	6	3
Number of errors in final position	5	N.T.	5	9	4	6	8	6	10	5	7	9	14	18	5	22	8	N.T.	N.T.	N.T.
Errors in initial position				1/t/	2/o/ 1/t/	2/o/ 2/k/ 1/dʒ/ 1/h/ 2/x/	4/p/ 1/x/	2/m/		1/o/ 3/p/ 1/m/			7/t/ 2/st/ 1/ʃ/ 2/x/	4/ʒ/ 2/n/ 2/k/ 1/t/ 1/dʒ/ 4/x/	2/s/ 3/t/ 1/dʒ/ 1/tʃ/ 5/x/	2/o/ 2/t/ 1/dʒ/ 1/ʃ/ 3/x/		3/o/ 1/j/ 1/w/ 1/ʒ/ 1/ʊ/ 1/l/	3/o/ 3/u/	3/o/
Errors in final position	2/o/ 1/x/		5/o/ 2/t/	7/o/ 2/t/	2/o/ 1/t/ 1/h/	4/o/ 2/k/	3/o/ 2/n/ 3/x/	3/o/ 3/t/	3/o/ 7/n/	3/o/ 2/ʊ/	4/o/ 3/f/	1/o/ 2/t/ 1/ð/ 1/h/ 1/f/ 3/x/	8/o/ 4/t/ 1/st/ 1/p/	8/o/ 2/t/ 2/ʃ/ 2/p/ 1/n/ 1/h/ 2/x/	2/o/ 3/x/	12/o/ 5/ʃ/ 1/t/ 4/x/	8/o/			

/o/ = omissions; / / = substitutions with sounds substituted; /x/ = distortions. N.T. = not tested.

substituted 7 times for the initial /b/, /t/ was substituted 10 times, in 3 instances for the initial /d/ and in 7 instances for the final /d/, and /k/ was substituted 5 times for the initial /g/. Amongst the partially-hearing children /t/ was substituted 3 times for /d/, 1 when /d/ was tested in the initial position and 2 when tested in the final position; /k/ was substituted 4 times for /g/, 2 when /g/ was tested in the initial position and 2 when tested in the final position.

Substitution involving changes both in the manner and in the place of articulation were also relatively frequent. For example, amongst the deaf children the nasal /m/ was produced twice in place of the initial /p/, /tʃ/ was produced twice in place of the initial /t/ and once in place of the final /k/. The semi-vowel /j/ was substituted once for the initial /t/, 3 times for the initial /d/, 6 times for the initial /k/ and 4 times for the initial /g/. Amongst the partially-hearing children /h/ was substituted once for the final /k/ and once for the initial /g/. The voiced affricative /dʒ/ was produced once in place of the initial /g/.

The most frequently distorted plosive consonant was final /p/. When produced it was accompanied by excessive breathiness. For example, /p/ as in 'ship' was heard as /pʰə/, [ʃɪpʰə].

Amongst the deaf children errors involving the plosive consonants amounted to approximately 32 per cent of their total consonant errors, whilst those of the partially-hearing children amounted to just over 17 per cent of their total consonant errors. The deaf children misarticulated nearly 67 per cent of all plosive consonants attempted, whilst the misarticulations of the partially-hearing children amounted to just over 13 per cent of all plosive consonants attempted.

Nasal consonants

In English there are normally three nasal consonants, /m/, /n/ and /ŋ/. In formation they are somewhat similar to the plosives, in that the oral occlusions are in the same places as for /p/, /t/ and /k/ respectively. They differ in two respects. The first way in which the nasals differ from the plosives is that whereas in the latter the obstruction to the breath emission is complete with the velum being closed, in the former the occlusion occurs only in the oral passage. Secondly, they are voiced continuants rather than plosives and as such have some of the characteristics of the vowels. Since the sounds are continuants, there must be some passage for the breath and the voice to escape. This passage is provided by dropping the velum, which ordinarily in speech is pressed against the back wall of the oral pharynx to close off the nasal passages, and forcing the breath or voice through the oral cavities. When the velum is dropped and the oral occlusion maintained, the nasal cavities are opened up so that the breath and voice go out through them.

The deaf children made 224 nasal consonant errors: of these 138 were omissions, 70 were substitutions and 16 distortions. The partially-hearing children made 31 nasal errors: 9 omissions, 18 substitutions and 4 distortions.

The deaf children omitted the final /ŋ/ 52 times. The initial /n/ was omitted 20 times whilst the final one was omitted 35 times. When tested initially /m/ was omitted 11 times and when tested finally 20 times. The partially-hearing children omitted final /ŋ/, final /n/ and final /m/ 3 times each.

Amongst the deaf children the most frequent substitution involved changes in the manner of articulation. For example, /p/ was produced 22 times in place of initial /m/, and /t/ 9 times in place of initial /n/. The above substitutions show that although the closure of the oral passage was correctly placed for the production of the nasals /n/ and /m/, the second prerequisite for the production of these consonants, that is, the dropping of the velum, was absent.

The partially-hearing children produced /p/ 4 times in place of initial /m/, and /t/ 3 times in place of final /n/. However, just over half of their substitutions in this consonant category involved changes in the place of articulation, for example, 2 productions of /n/ in place of /m/ and vice versa. Moreover, /n/ was produced 7 times in place of /ŋ/.

The most commonly distorted nasal consonant was /m/ as in 'moon' and 'farm'. This phoneme was mainly given as a strongly nasalised /m/ with some overtones of /b/, the words 'farm' and 'moon', for example, being heard as [faːmᵇə] and [mᵇun] respectively.

Amongst the deaf children errors involving the nasal consonants accounted for nearly 17 per cent of their total consonant errors, whilst those of the partially-hearing children accounted for approximately 14 per cent of their total consonant errors. The deaf children misarticulated nearly 77 per cent of all nasal consonants attempted whilst the partially-hearing children misarticulated approximately 23 per cent of all nasal consonants attempted.

Fricative consonants

Many of the sounds of speech are produced not by complete but by partial obstruction of the breath emission, so that what is heard is the friction or hissing as the breath passes through the narrow opening, hence the term 'fricative'. Each sound so produced with only the friction of the breath has its counterpart in another sound produced in like manner but with the addition of the voice.

The deaf children made 466 fricative consonant errors; of these 268 were omissions, 167 substitutions and 31 distortions. The partially-hearing children made 103 fricative errors: 27 omissions, 55 substitutions and 19 distortions. Both the deaf and the partially-hearing children found the sibilants /s/, /z/ and /ʃ/ most difficult to produce. The deaf children omitted /s/ 57 times (17 times in the initial position and 40 times in the final position), /z/ 69 times (22 times in the initial position and 47 times in the final position) and /ʃ/ 56 times (20 times in the initial position and 36 times in the final position). Amongst the partially-hearing children the three most frequently omitted fricative consonants were the final /z/ (8 times), the final /s/ (8 times) and the final /v/ (4 times).

The plosive consonants /t/ and /p/ were the most frequently substituted phonemes for the fricative consonants. For example, among the deaf children /p/ was substituted 13 times for the initial /f/, /t/ was substituted 26 times for the initial /s/, 16 times for the initial /ʃ/, 8 times for the initial /f/ and 7 times for the final /θ/. Amongst the partially-hearing /p/ was substituted 3 times for the initial /f/ and twice for the final /z/, /t/ was substituted 7 times for the initial /s/ and 4 times for the final /s/, once for the initial /z/ and twice for the final /z/ and 3 times for the initial /ʃ/.

Another frequent substitution error was the interchange of the sibilants. For example, amongst the deaf children /ʃ/ was produced 3 times in place of /s/ and 6 times in place of /z/, /s/ was produced twice in place of /z/, /ʒ/ was produced 5 times in place of /z/ and 4 times in place of /ʃ/. Amongst the partially-hearing children /ʃ/ was produced once in place of /s/ and twice in place of /z/, /s/ was produced twice in place of /ʃ/ and /ʒ/ was produced 4 times in place of /z/.

The three most frequently distorted fricative consonants among the deaf children were /s/, /ʃ/ and /θ/. Distortion of /s/ when tested initially was mainly due to intrusive overtones of the plosive consonant /t/. For example, the word 'sun' was heard as [sᵗʌn]. Distortion of final /s/ was mainly due to excessive prolongation followed by a sudden release of breath. For example, the word 'house' was heard as [haʊsʲᵊ]. Distortion of /ʃ/ was similar in nature. For example, the word 'ship' was heard as [ʃᵗɪp] and sometimes as [ʃʰɪp]. Distortion involving /θ/ was mainly due to a partial arrest of the continuous flow of breath required for its production. For example, the word 'bath' was heard as [baᵗθ]. In some instances /θ/ was followed by an abrupt release of breath: [baᵗθᵊ]. Amongst the partially-hearing the most frequently distorted fricative consonants were /ʃ/, which was most commonly heard as /ʃʰᵊ/ as in [fɪʃʰᵊ], and /z/ which was heard as /ᵗz/ as in [ᵗzu].

Nearly 35 per cent of the total consonant errors of the deaf children were associated with the fricative consonants. Amongst the partially-hearing, errors involving the fricative consonants amounted to just over 44 per cent of their total consonant errors.

When the above errors were expressed as percentages of total possible errors it was found that the deaf children misarticulated a little over 80 per cent of all fricative consonants attempted whilst the partially-hearing misarticulated 37·4 per cent of all fricative consonants attempted.

Other consonants

This category consists of the affricative consonant /tʃ/, the lateral consonant /l/, the rolled sound /r/, the glottal fricative /h/ and the semi-vowel /w/. The deaf children made 221 errors under this consonant category. Of these 144 were omissions, 57 were substitutions and the remaining 20 distortions. The partially-hearing children made 57 errors under this consonant category. Of these 31 were omissions, 19 were substitutions and the remaining 7 were distortions.

Amongst the deaf children the three most frequently omitted phonemes in this consonant category were the initial /h/ (35 times), the affricative /tʃ/ (34 times when tested in the final position and 19 times when tested in the initial position) and the final /l/ (30 times). Amongst the partially-hearing children /tʃ/ was omitted 14 times (2 initially and 12 finally), and final /l/ 8 times. The phonemes /r/, /w/ and /h/ were omitted 3 times each.

The most frequently substituted phonemes for the affricative /tʃ/ were the fricative consonants /t/ and /ʃ/. For example, the deaf children produced /t/ 5 times and /ʃ/ twice in place of the initial /tʃ/, and /ʃ/ 5 times in place of the final /tʃ/. The partially-hearing children produced /t/ twice and /ʃ/ once in place of the initial /tʃ/, and /ʃ/ 5 times and /t/ once in place of the final /tʃ/.

The most common substitutions among the deaf children for /r/, /w/ and /h/ were the plosive consonants /t/ and /p/ and the fricative consonant /v/. The partially-hearing children produced /v/ 3 times in place of /w/, and the consonants /j/, /w/, /ʒ/, /v/ and /l/ were produced once each in place of the initial /r/.

The phoneme /tʃ/ was the only one distorted in this consonant category. Distortions of this consonant when tested in the initial position were mainly due to an abrupt release of its plosive component. Thus the test word 'chair' was heard as [tᵊʃɛə]. Distortion of final /tʃ/ was mainly due to excessive prolongation of its second component followed by a sudden release of breath. For example, the test word 'watch' was heard as [wɔtʃːʰə].

Amongst the deaf children errors involving the above consonants amounted to 16·52 per cent of their total consonant errors, while those made by the partially-hearing amounted to nearly 25 per cent of their total consonant errors. The deaf children misarticulated 63·48 per cent of all the above consonants attempted, whilst the partially-hearing misarticulated a little over 35 per cent of all the above consonants attempted.

THE 1980 STUDY

Three groups of hearing-impaired children, the great majority drawn from a single school, participated in this investigation. The main difference between the three groups of children was their type of audiogram configuration (Figure 3.5). Group A, consisting of 11 children (7 boys and 4 girls) and with an average age of 11·3 years (range 10·2 years to 12·8 years) exhibited symmetrical bilateral hearing losses with a 'sloping' pure tone audiogram configuration (hearing deteriorating at the rate of 15 to 20 dB per octave from 250 Hz to 4000 Hz). Group B, consisting of 9 children (5 boys and 4 girls) and with an average age of 11·6 years (range 10·4 years to 13·3 years) also had symmetrical bilateral hearing losses but in this case the audiogram configuration of each child was of the 'flat' type (hearing levels at 250, 500, 2000 and 4000 Hz within ±20 dB of the hearing level at 1000 Hz). Group C consisted of 8 children (4 boys and 4 girls). Their average age was 10·9 years (range 9·8 years to 12·7 years) and their type of audiogram configuration was a combination of the two types characterising the children in groups A and B – hearing levels steadily falling from 250 Hz to 1000 Hz and thereafter, up to 4000 Hz, remaining relatively the same. In terms of average hearing levels in dB (averaged across the main audiometric frequencies 250 Hz to 4000 Hz), all three groups of children had similar hearing losses ranging from 67·0 dB to 71·4 dB.

As far as could be ascertained onset of deafness among the children taking part was either from birth or during the first year of life. All the children were experienced hearing aid users and at the time of testing most of them were fitted with similar binaural ear-level hearing aids.

The articulation test used was constructed by the writer and it consisted of 27 monosyllabic words which were specially selected (a) to be within the vocabulary of the children involved and (b) to test a representative number of vowels, diphthongs and consonants in the English language.

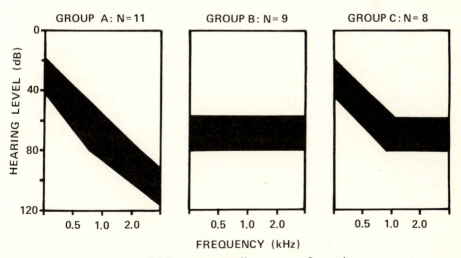

FIGURE 3.5 Pure tone audiogram configuration

Table 3.5 shows the words selected together with the phonemes tested in each word: 11 vowels and 4 diphthongs were tested in the medial position while the same 16 consonants were tested both in the initial and final position. Each word was represented pictorially on a separate 6 cm × 8 cm card. The responses of the children were put on magnetic tape and later on transcribed phonetically. The misarticulations observed were assigned to the same categories as used in the first study.

VOWEL AND DIPHTHONG ERRORS

The children in group A made 23 vowel and diphthong errors, an average of 2·07 errors per child; the children in group B made 14 errors, on average

TABLE 3.5   Articulation test

	Phonemes tested		
Word	initially (I)	medially (M)	finally (F)
1 pig	p	ɪ	g
2 ship	ʃ		p
3 boy	b	ɔɪ	
4 ball		ɔ	
5 bath			θ
6 book		ʊ	k
7 cat	k	æ	t
8 dog	d	ɒ	
9 red		ɛ	d
10 gun	g	ʌ	n
11 chair	tʃ	ɛə	
12 watch			tʃ
13 moon	m	u	
14 farm		ɑ	m
15 knife	n	aɪ	f
16 fish			ʃ
17 house		aʊ	s
18 sun	s		
19 girl		ɜ	
20 five	f		v
21 ten	t		
22 keys		i	z
23 zoo	z		
24 tub			b
25 vest	v		
26 thief	θ		
27 judge	dʒ		dʒ

of 1·55 errors per child; and the children in group C made 16 errors, an average of 2·00 errors per child. For groups A and C these errors amounted to nearly 14 per cent of all vowels and diphthongs attempted, whilst for group B, the errors made amounted to just over 10 per cent (Table 3.6). The differences observed in favour of group B ('flat' hearing impairment) proved to be statistically significant at the 10 per cent level.

It can be noted that category 3 (vowel prolongation) included the greatest number of errors made by the hearing-impaired children in groups A and C. For group B the greatest number of errors were in category 2 (vowel neutralisation). The number of errors in the remaining two vowel error categories was very small and the group differences observed were non-significant. The children in group A made on average significantly ($p=0.05$) more diphthong errors than the children in the other two groups.

The actual vowel and diphthong errors made by the children are shown in Table 3.7. Two outstanding error features common to all the children emerge from this table. The first one relates to the high incidence of neutralisation and the second one to the high incidence of excessive prolongation affecting both pure vowels and diphthongs.

Prolongation affecting diphthongs produced two types of error. The most common mistake was to prolong excessively the first component of the diphthong with its second component being omitted. For example, /aɪ/ as in 'knife' was heard as /aː/, [naː] with or without the final /f/. The second type of error again involved the excessive prolongation of the first component of the glide but on this occasion the diphthong was heard as two distinct vowels. For example, the diphthong /ɛə/ as in 'chair' was heard as /ɛːə/, [tʃɛːə].

TABLE 3.6   Vowel and diphthong errors

	Average number of errors		
Error categories	Group A (N=11 children)	Group B (N=9 children)	Group C (N=8 children)
1 Substitution	0·09		0·12
2 Neutralisation	0·54	0·66	0·60
3 Prolongation	0·72	0·33	0·72
4 Diphthongisation	0·09	0·11	0·12
5 Diphthong errors	0·63	0·44	0·50
Total vowel and diphthong errors	2·07 (13·93%)	1·55 (10·37%)	2·00 (13·33%)

TABLE 3.7 Vowel and diphthong errors

Groups	i	ɪ	ɛ	æ	ɑ	ʌ	ɜ	ɒ	ɔ	ʊ	u	aʊ	ɔɪ	ɛə
A: Number of errors	1	2	1	1		2	2	2	1	2	2	2	1	3
B: Number of errors	1	1	1		2	1	1	1	1	1	1	1		2
C: Number of errors		2		1	1	1	1	1	1	1	2	1		2
Total number of errors	**2**	**5**	**2**	**2**	**3**	**4**	**4**	**4**	**3**	**4**	**5**	**4**	**1**	**7**
A: Type of error	1/ə/ 2/i/		1/ə/ 1/ə/	1/ə/		2/ə/	1/ɜː/ 1/ə/	1/ɒɪ/ 1/ɔː/	1/ɔː/ 1/ə/	1/ə/ 1/u/	2/uː/	1/ə/ 1/aː/	1/ə/	2/ɜː/ 1/ə/
B: Type of error	1/ə/ 1/ə/				2/ə/	1/ə/	1/ɜː/	1/ɒɪ/	1/ɔː/	1/ə/	1/uː/	1/aɪ/	1/ɔː/	2/ɜː/
C: Type of error	1/i/ 1/ɪə/	1/ə/		1/ə/	1/ə/	1/ə/	1/ɜː/	1/ə/	1/ɔː/	1/u/	2/uː/	1/ə/	1/ɔɪ/	1/ɛə/ 1/ɜː/

CONSONANT ERRORS

The children in group A ($N=11$) made 110 consonant errors, 31 per cent of all consonants attempted (Table 3.10). Of these errors, 47, an average of 4·27 errors per child were associated with initial consonants (Table 3.8), whilst the remaining 63, an average of 5·72 errors per child were associated with final consonants (Table 3.9). The respective average errors for the other two groups of children were not significantly different from those quoted above. Note that for all children errors involving the final consonants were more numerous than errors involving the initial consonants. The most numerous errors affecting initial consonants for all three groups of children were errors of substitution. For final consonants they were errors of distortion.

Omissions and distortions of final consonants were much more

TABLE 3.8   Consonant errors (initial position)

Error categories	Average number of errors		
	Group A ($N=11$)	Group B ($N=9$)	Group C ($N=8$)
Plosives			
Omissions	0·27		0·37
Substitutions	0·45	0·44	0·25
Distortions		0·11	
Nasals			
Omissions			
Substitutions	0·36	0·11	0·25
Distortions		0·22	0·12
Fricatives			
Omissions	0·09		0·12
Substitutions	1·54	1·21	1·12
Distortions	0·54	0·77	0·87
Affricatives			
Omissions	0·18	0·33	0·37
Substitutions	0·81	0·44	0·62
Distortions		0·33	0·25
All initial consonants			
Omissions (O)	0·54	0·33	0·86
Substitutions (S)	3·18	2·20	2·24
Distortions (D)	0·54	1·43	1·24
O+S+D	4·27	4·00	4·34
	(26·70%)	(25·00%)	(26·94%)

TABLE 3.9   Consonant errors (final position)

	Average number of errors		
Error categories	Group A (N=11)	Group B (N=9)	Group C (N=8)
Plosives			
Omissions	0·54	0·55	0·87
Substitutions	0·54	0·55	0·12
Distortions	0·45	0·66	0·72
Nasals			
Omissions	0·45	0·22	0·24
Substitutions			0·12
Distortions	0·18	0·11	0·12
Fricatives			
Omissions	0·81	0·66	1·00
Substitutions	0·63	0·66	0·50
Distortions	0·72	0·66	0·72
Affricatives			
Omissions	0·27	0·44	0·36
Substitutions			0·12
Distortions	1·09	0·88	0·87
All final consonants			
Omissions (O)	2·09	1·87	2·50
Substitutions (S)	1·18	1·21	0·87
Distortions (D)	2·45	2·31	2·50
O+S+D	5·72	5·44	5·87
	(35·79%)	(34·02%)	(36·71%)

numerous than omissions and distortions of initial consonants for all
three groups of children. Consonant substitutions showed the opposite
picture, substitution errors being more numerous with the initial
consonants than with the final consonants, and again this was true for all
three groups of children. When both initial and final errors were
combined it was found that on average the children in group A made
more substitution errors ($p=0·05$) than the children in either of the other
two groups (Table 3.10). In all other consonant error categories the
differences between the three groups of children were small and none
proved to be statistically significant.

No attempt will be made here to describe in detail the actual consonant
errors made by each group of children. This information is summarised in
Tables 3.11 and 3.12. Suffice it to state that all three groups of children
experienced the same order of difficulty in the production of consonants.

TABLE 3.10   Consonant and vowel errors

	Average number of errors		
Error categories	Group A (N=11)	Group B (N=9)	Group C (N=8)
All consonants			
(Initial and final)			
Omissions (O)	2·63	2·22	3·37
Substitutions (S)	4·36	3·33	3·12
Distortions (D)	3·00	3·88	3·70
O+S+D	10·00	9·37	10·19
	(31·25%)	(29·50%)	(31·82%)
Total vowel and			
consonant errors	12·07	10·92	12·19
	(25·70%)	(23·23%)	(25·94%)

For both initial and final consonants, for example, the children in each group experienced more difficulty with the pronunciation of the affricatives followed by the fricatives, then the nasals and finally the plosives.

When both vowel and consonant errors were combined (Table 3.10) it was found that the children in groups A and C made on average 12 errors per child while the children in group B made on average 11 errors per child. In other words the children in each group misarticulated nearly a quarter of all phonemes attempted (Figure 3.6). The small differences observed between groups did not prove statistically significant.

INTEGRATION

In the first study the deaf children misarticulated nearly 56 per cent of all vowels and diphthongs attempted, whilst the partially-hearing children misarticulated approximately 9 per cent of all vowels and diphthongs attempted. The vowel and diphthong errors of the children in the second study varied from 10 per cent to 14 per cent and these figures compare favourably with the 9 per cent errors exhibited by the partially-hearing children in the first study. This was expected mainly because the mean hearing levels of the partially-hearing children in both studies were of similar magnitude.

In both studies vowel substitution and vowel neutralisation were common articulatory mistakes in the speech of the children. According to Angelocci, Kopp and Holbrook (1964) these errors can be explained by the fact that deaf talkers exhibit a much more limited range of frequencies

TABLE 3.11 Consonant errors (initial position)

	Plosives						Nasals		Fricatives						Affricatives	
	p	b	t	d	k	g	m	n	f	v	θ	s	z	ʃ	tʃ	dʒ
A: Number of errors	1			1	2	4	3	1	3	3	5	5	5	3	4	7
B: Number of errors				1	1	3	2	1	2	3	3	3	3	4	4	6
C: Number of errors				1	2	2	2	1	3	2	2	4	3	3	5	5
Total number of errors	**1**			**3**	**5**	**9**	**7**	**3**	**8**	**8**	**10**	**12**	**11**	**10**	**13**	**18**
A: Type of error	1/t/			1/t/	1/o/ 1/t/	2/o/ 1/k/ 1/h/	3/p/	1/t/	1/o/ 1/t/ 1/p/	2/f/ 1/fʲ/	3/t/ 2/θʲ/	3/t/ 1/sʲ/ 1/f/	3/ʒ/ 1/t/ 1/tz/	1/tʃ/ 1/s/ 1/dʒ/	2/t/ 2/ʃ/	3/d/ 1/t/ 2/o/ 1/ʃ/
B: Type of error				1/t/	1/t/	2/k/ 1/o/	1/p/ 1/mᵇ/	1/nᵗ/	1/m/ 1/p/	1/f/ 1/b/ 1/t/	1/t/ 1/ð/ 1/θᵗ/	1/ʃ/ 1/ʃʲ/ 1/sʲ/	2/ʒ/ 1/tᶻ/	2/tʃ/ 1/tˢ/ 1/f/	2/t/ 2/ʃ/	3/o/ 1/h/ 1/tʃ/ 1/ʃ/
C: Type of error				1/t/	2/o/	1/o/ 1/d/	1/b/ 1/mᵇ/	1/t/	1/o/ 1/fʰ/ 1/t/	1/f/ 1/t/	1/t/ 1/θt/	3/t/ 1/st/	2/ᵛz/ 1/ʃ/	2/ˢʃ/ 1/ʒ/	3/ʃ/ 2/ˢʃ/	3/o/ 1/ʒ/ 1/t/

/o/ omission

TABLE 3.12 Consonant errors (final position)

Groups	Plosives						Nasals		Fricatives						Affricatives	
	p	b	t	d	k	g	m	n	f	v	θ	s	z	ʃ	tʃ	dʒ
A: Number of errors	2	2	3	4	3	3	4	3	2	3	4	6	7	2	7	8
B: Number of errors	1	2	3	5	2	3	2	1	2	3	2	4	5	2	6	6
C: Number of errors	1	2	3	3	2	3	2	2	2	3	3	3	5	2	5	6
Total number of errors	**4**	**6**	**9**	**12**	**7**	**9**	**8**	**6**	**6**	**9**	**9**	**13**	**17**	**6**	**18**	**20**
A: Type of error	1/k/ 1/p^{hə}/	2/b^{hə}/	1/o/ 1/ts/ 1/ʃ/	2/o/ 2/t/	1/o/ 1/t/ 1/k^{hə}/	2/o/ 1/k/	3/o/ 1/m^{bə}/	2/o/ 1/n^{ə}/	1/o/ 1/f^{ə}/ 1/fʃ/	1/o/ 1/f^{ə}/ 1/fʃ/	1/o/ 1/t^{ə}/ 1/θ^{ə}/	4/o/ 1/ʃ/ 1/ʃ^{hə}/	5/ʃ/ 2/o/	2/o/ 2/ʃ^{hə}/	7/ʃ^{h}/	3/o/ 5/ʃ^{hə}/
B: Type of error	1/p^{hə}/ 1/p/	1/h^{ə}/ 1/p/	1/p/ 1/o/ 1/ʃs/	2/o/ 1/t/ 1/tʃ/ 1/də/	1/o/ 1/k^{hə}/	1/o/ 1/t/ 1/gh^{ə}/	1/o/ 1/m^{bə}/	1/o/	1/o/ 1/fʃ/	2/o/ 1/ʃ/	1/tθ/ 1/tθ^{ə}/	2/o/ 1/ʃ^{hə}/ 1/ʃ/	1/o/ 4/ʃ/	1/o/ 2/ʃ^{hə}/	6/ʃ:/	4/o/ 1/ʃ^{hə}/ 1/tʃ^{hə}/
C: Type of error	1/p^{hə}/	2/b^{hə}/	2/o/ 1/tʃ/	2/o/ 1/d^{ə}/	1/o/ 1/t/	2/o/ 1/gh^{ə}/	1/m^{ə}/ 1/o/	1/o/ 1/t/	1/o/ 1/fʃ/	2/o/ 1/fʃ/	1/t^{ə}θ/ 1/o/ 1/θ^{tə}/	2/o/ 1/ʃ^{tə}/1	3/ʃʃ/	3/o/ 2/'ʃ^{ə}/ 1/ʃʃ/	5/ʃ:/	3/o/ 2/'ʃ^{ə}/ 1/ʃʃ/

/o/ omission

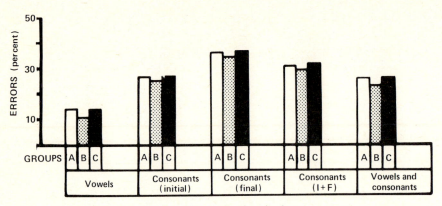

FIGURE 3.6 Distribution of articulatory errors

between the first two formants* than seen in normal talkers. In other words they found that the formants of the vowels produced by deaf children tended to group together, approaching the pattern for the neutral /ə/ vowel. This ties in with the results already reported that many of the vowel substitutions were towards the neutral vowel. According to Angelocci and his associates these articulatory errors were brought about because the deaf children did not use efficiently the extremes of their oral cavity with their tongue movements, thus exhibiting inaccuracy of tongue placement and configuration.

Both the deaf and the partially-hearing children experienced considerable difficulty in the production of diphthongs and this is in line with the findings of Hudgins and Numbers (1942). The predominant mistake here involved the movement of the tongue from the position of the first component of the glide to the position necessary for the production of the second component of the glide. The tongue movement was either too slow, resulting in the two components of the glide being perceived as two separate vowels or incomplete, thus resulting in the non-production of the second component of the glide. These misarticulations together with vowel prolongation are essentially distortions involving the durational characteristics of phonemes (Levitt, 1971; Monsen, 1974, 1978).

In general the vowel errors described here are similar to those reported in other studies, indicating that vowels with low tongue position are more easily produced than those with mid or high tongue position (Nober, 1967; Smith, 1973; Geffner and Freeman, 1980). According to Boone

* When a speaker produces vowel sounds the sound energy radiated from his lips is concentrated into relatively narrow bands of frequencies. These bands of strong energy are called formants and they are brought about by the resonant characteristics of the vocal tract. The formants are numbered in ascending order of frequency: the first formant ($F1$) is the formant of lowest frequency and $F2$, $F3$, etc. are higher frequency formants. The fundamental frequency which gives rise to the pitch of voice is referred to as Fo.

(1966) this is due to the fact that deaf children tend to keep their tongues too far back and too low in the mouth, thus interfering with the production of front and high vowels. Table 3.13 shows the vowels and diphthongs in rank order of difficulty as reported in several studies.

With regard to consonant errors the deaf children in the first study misarticulated nearly 72 per cent of all consonants attempted whilst the partially-hearing children misarticulated a little over 26 per cent of all consonants attempted. In the 1980 study the relevant percentage figures varied from 29·5 to nearly 32 per cent.

Amongst the deaf children omission errors were more numerous, followed by substitutions and finally by distortions. Amongst the partially-hearing children in both studies substitution errors were more numerous with omissions and distortions closely following. Both deaf and partially-hearing children misarticulated final consonants more frequently than initial consonants.

With both groups of children (deaf and partially-hearing) omission errors were more numerous with final consonants while substitutions were more numerous with initial consonants, a finding that is in agreement with that of Carlin (1964), Nober (1967) and Smith (1973). In

TABLE 3.13   Vowels and diphthongs: rank order of difficulty
(from the most difficult to the most easy)

Hudgins & Numbers (1942) Deaf	Markides (1967) Deaf	Markides (1967) Partially-hearing	Markides (1980b) Partially-hearing	Geffner & Freeman (1980) Deaf
	εə	εə	εə	
aɪ	ʌ	ɪ	u	ɪ
ɔɪ	aɪ	u	ɪ	oʊ
3	ɒ	aɪ	aɪ	ɔɪ
i	æ	ʌ	ʊ	ɔ
ɛ	ɛ	ɔ	ɒ	ɛ
ɒ	ɪ	ɔɪ	3	ɑ
ʊ	3	ɑ	ʌ	
oʊ				ɪʊ
u	ɔɪ	ɒ	ɔɪ	aɪ
aʊ	i	ʊ	ɔ	aʊ
ɪ	ʊ	i	ɑ	æ
eɪ				
ɔ	ɔ	ɛ	æ	u
æ	u	æ	i	ʌ
u				
ɑ	ɑ	3	ɛ	ɛ
ʌ	aʊ	aʊ	aʊ	

contrast Hudgins and Numbers (1942) and Geffner and Freeman (1980) found omission of initial consonants was more frequent than omission of final consonants. According to the latter authors this difference in error analysis may reflect differences in sampling and test materials employed.

Of more immediate interest here are the types of articulatory errors made by the children. A high proportion of them were basically errors of durational character. One of the principal consequences of this involved the dysfunction of voiced and voiceless cognates. In normal speech, voiceless plosives should be produced with a longer closure duration than their voiced cognates. Furthermore, there should be a lag of 50 to 100 ms between release of closure and onset of voicing with voiceless plosives, whereas with voiced stops voicing should precede or perhaps be coincident with the release of closure (Hutchinson and Smith, 1980). Often the relative durational aspects of pressure release and voicing onsets are inaccurate among hearing-impaired children resulting in

TABLE 3.14   Consonants: rank order of difficulty (from the most difficult to the most easy)

Hudgins & Numbers (1942) Deaf	Markides (1967) Deaf	Markides (1967) Partially-hearing	Markides (1980b) Partially-hearing	Geffner & Freeman (1980) Deaf
dʒ			dʒ	ŋ
d	ŋ	z	tʃ	g
h	s	tʃ	z	z
b	ʃ	s	s	dʒ
g	z	ŋ	θ	tʃ
ʃ	g	ʃ	g	k
l	k	θ	v	s
r	d	r	ʃ	ʃ
tʃ	tʃ	l	m	θ
j				t
z	n	v	d	j
s	m	g	f	n
θ	v	m		d
w	h	w		r
ʌ				m
t	θ	f		h
ʃ	f	d		ð
ð				l
k	t	n	k	v
v	r	k	n	w
ŋ	w	h		
p	l	t	t	f
n	p	p	b	p
m	b	b	p	b

difficulties regarding the voiced–voiceless dysfunction (Calvert, 1964; Monsen, 1976; Hutchinson and Smith, 1976).

A large number of consonant errors were brought about predominantly as a result of poor control over the manner and place of articulation. Improper control of the velum for example, caused nasalisation of both vowels and consonants; ineffective closure in the production of plosives brought about distortion, intrusions or substitutions. Similar articulatory errors were also associated with incorrect placement of the tongue especially in the production of fricatives.

The visibility of phonemes proved to be an important factor affecting the articulatory skills of both deaf and partially-hearing children. All relevant studies (Nober, 1967; Smith, 1973; Geffner and Freeman, 1980) reported unanimously that bilabials and labiodentals were produced more correctly than palatals and fricatives, affricates, and glottals. Table 3.14 shows more detailed information regarding the rank order of difficulty of consonants as reported in various studies.

CHAPTER FOUR

Prosodic features

Prosodic or suprasegmental features are usually either listed as the set of features consisting of pitch, stress and quantity (Hamp, 1957) or defined as those that are 'overlaid' on the inherent features of the individual phonetic segment. Strictly speaking the two terms (prosodic, suprasegmental) are not synonymous. Some prosodic aspects of speech such as duration and quantity, for example, relate both to the segmental and the suprasegmental elements of speech. In this book both terms will be used interchangeably. Conventionally there are three prosodic aspects important to English: (*a*) intonation, (*b*) duration and quantity, and (*c*) stress and emphasis.

Prosodic cues are very important in the perception of speech and this was most ably highlighted by an experiment carried out by Kozhevnikov and Christovich in 1965. They presented short phrases to subjects through a narrow filter with a passband from 906 to 1141 Hz, which made the speech unintelligible by removing the cues to place of articulation. The subjects involved attempted to identify the phrases, guessing where necessary. Word accent was incorrect in only 3 per cent of 2617 words given as responses, though overall phrase intelligibility was only 30 per cent. It might be argued that this result was not surprising, since the necessary information about pitch and timing was passed by the filter – *but this is precisely the point*. Prosodic features are transmitted, even when the speech is unrecognisable, provided enough information on syllabicity is presented. According to Huggins (1972) prosodic features are the most resistant parts of the speech waveform to any naturally occurring form of distortion and for this reason alone it would be most surprising if prosodic cues were not fundamental in the perception of running speech. As might be anticipated, prosodic features are very often disturbed in the speech of hearing-impaired children.

The most common errors affecting the prosodic aspects of the speech of deaf children relate to intonation, breath control, rate of speaking, phrasing and pausing, rhythm and stress and voice quality.

INTONATION

Intonation is perhaps the most complex of the prosodic features. It refers primarily to variation in fundamental frequency which functions at the phrase or sentence level and imparts semantic and syntactic information. For example, in English declarative sentences are characterised by a terminal decrease in Fo and questions are often stated with a terminal increase in Fo. Amongst hearing-impaired children intonation is usually flat and monotonous (Hood and Dixon, 1949) and this according to Angelocci, Kopp and Holbrook (1964) and Mártony (1968), is due to the fact that deaf children cannot control or have very limited control over their voice frequency, particularly with vowels of long duration.

BREATH CONTROL

Deaf speakers as a rule not only produce sound inefficiently but also pause for breath more frequently. Among the first workers to emphasise the importance of breath control were Haycock (1933), Voelker (1935), Scuri (1935), Mason and Bright (1937), and Hudgins (1946). They found that deaf subjects used short, irregular breath groups of only one or two words in length and that inappropriate pauses for breath interrupted the natural flow of speech thus affecting intelligibility. A common source of difficulty noted was the excessive expenditure of breath on single syllables.

In 1970 Holm stated that the valvic action of the larynx of deaf children during speech is impaired and sometimes it is not even developed. He found the mean air flow of deaf children while speaking to be three times the similar flow of normal children and he was of the opinion that the laryngeal structures of deaf children, especially those anatomical parts that are prominent during speech, were not properly developed. In particular he stated that the laryngeal development at the level of the vocal folds of a deaf child of 2·5 years was equivalent to that of a normal child of 6 months, and that of a deaf child of 6 years resembled that of a normal child of 2 or 2·5 years. In view of these anatomical differences he surmised that the deaf child has poor control over his vocal folds especially when maintaining tension in them. This affects the deaf child's ability in maintaining an adequate acoustic energy with the result that the voice produced is excessively breathy with inappropriate interruptions. Similar results were more recently put forward by Hutchinson and Smith (1976), Forner and Hixon (1977) and Hutchinson, Kornhauser, Beasley and Beasley (1978). Another voice quality problem that is directly associated with inappropriate control of laryngeal valving is tension or harshness. Generally speaking deaf children speak with lung volumes well below normal capacity thus necessitating excessive muscular activity to maintain an acceptable level of pressure. This excessive activity of the laryngeal muscles can bring about the perceptual consequence of tension or harshness.

RHYTHM AND STRESS

Closely allied to the problem of breath control, which affects phrasing directly, is that of proper rhythm and stress. The importance of rhythm and stress was realised a long time ago (Story, 1915; Bell, 1916; Haycock, 1933). Haycock in particular emphasised that it was not enough to teach deaf children to articulate single sounds correctly, or even to produce clear patterns of individual words but 'it is only when we treat a sentence as a synthetic whole, that rhythmic speech is realisable'. Hudgins and Numbers (1942) found a high correlation between rhythmic errors and poor intelligibility. Sentences that were either arhythmic or had incorrect rhythm were also the least intelligible of the sentences studied. Hudgins (1946) found that poor respiratory control leads not only to incorrect grouping of syllables, but also to improper placing of stress. A more recent study by John and Howarth (1965) demonstrated the important contribution of rhythm to speech intelligibility. They noted that the speech of deaf children exhibited a high proportion of errors relating to faulty time relationships. In particular they noted little continuity from sound to sound or from word to word within an utterance thus resulting in faulty operation of a stress pattern. By concentrating their teaching solely on the temporal aspects of speech they achieved a great improvement in speech intelligibility. Another important variable controlling the placing of stress is the relative duration of stressed and unstressed syllables (Ando and Canter, 1969). We have already seen that many deaf children distort the duration of most vowels and consonants by prolonging their average durations by three or four times that of normal hearing children. In addition there are abnormalities in the relative durational aspects of phonemes in sequence (Calvert, 1964). These time distortions tend to interfere with and sometimes destroy completely the rhythmic aspects of speech. Under these conditions, even if all phonemes are correctly identified, the listener may find it very difficult to follow the spoken message.

PAUSING

Defective breath control and durational abnormalities bring about inappropriate pausing which affects directly the rate of speaking. In 1964

Calvert reported that deaf speakers tended to interpose a pause between the juncture of two syllables and in 1969 Ando and Canter stated that this exaggerated use of internal open juncture between syllables contributed to a slow rate of speech which in turn affected stress and emphasis (stress on the sentence level) and distorted rhythm.

An abnormal amount of pausing in the speech of deaf children has been noted by several workers. Voelker (1935), for example, stated that deaf subjects exhibited pausing between utterances which were four times longer than the maximum pausing of normal speakers. Hardy, Pauls and Haskins (1958) noted a higher incidence of pauses in the speech of partially-hearing children than in the speech of normal hearing children. John and Howarth (1965) stated that silences between words often accounted for half the time a hearing-impaired child took to say a sentence.

RATE OF SPEAKING

It is generally agreed that the overall rate of speech is slower in the deaf (Colton and Cooker, 1968). As far back as 1934 Hudgins described the speech of deaf children as slow and laboured. The same observations were also made by Haycock (1933) when he expressed the opinion that the reasons for this slow rate of speaking was due not only to faulty breath control and exaggerated articulation of individual phonemes but also to faulty speech teaching methods that emphasised the production of isolated words instead of concentrating on the rhythmic production of phrases and sentences. Hood (1966) reported that deaf speakers took twice as long and sometimes three and a half times as long to say a particular sentence as normal hearing speakers.

VOICE QUALITY

In addition to problems of intonation, breath control, rate of speaking, rhythm and stress, many deaf children also tend to have severe difficulties with voice quality. An unpleasant voice quality, particularly when it is associated with an abnormally high pitch, is a formidable impediment to communication. Angelocci, Kopp and Holbrook (1964) and more recently Mártony (1968) have shown that a large number of deaf children exhibit on average a higher voice pitch than normal hearing children. Many deaf children also tend to expend a lot of energy in producing speech and this leads to a voice quality known as 'overfortis'. Other common problems in voice quality among hearing-impaired children include excessive breathiness, due to improper control of the closing of the vocal cords, nasality, due to improper control of the velum, stridency, due to improper control of intensity, and harshness primarily due to excessive laryngeal muscle activity.

A considerable amount of the information presented so far in this chapter derived from experimental work involving careful analysis of the speech of deaf children. In addition to this, however, it would be of interest to know how the professional person himself, and also the man in the street, perceives and categorises some of the prosodic features of the speech of deaf children. Such information was collected by the writer in 1967 and more recently in 1980. The results obtained are summarised in the rest of this chapter.

SPEECH RATINGS

The information obtained in 1967 related to 85 pupils, 58 deaf and 27 partially-hearing. The more recent information (1980a) was obtained in a study of the speech of 28 partially-hearing children. The relevant information on the children in these two studies has already been presented in the previous chapter.

In both studies the children involved were required to describe a set of colourful unrelated pictures, their responses being recorded on magnetic tape for later assessment regarding voice quality, pitch, loudness, intonation and rate of speaking. In the first study the speech of each child was assessed by two panels of judges consisting of three persons each. The first judges were the teachers of the children – experienced listeners. The second panel consisted of people who were totally naive with regard to speech of deaf children – inexperienced listeners. The judges were not the same for all the children. Altogether 30 teachers of the deaf and 36 lay people acted as judges. In the second study the assessment of each child's speech was carried out by the class teacher.

In both studies each judge was given a special form (Figure 4.1) and was requested to listen to the speech of each child and then indicate his or her rating with regard to voice quality, pitch, loudness, intonation and rate of speaking.

The ratings obtained in both studies are presented in Tables 4.1–10. In the first study the ratings of each group of judges were first treated separately and then combined. When summarising the ratings of each group of judges, under 'partial agreement' (PA) were placed all the children where two out of three judges were in agreement, and under 'full agreement' (FA) were placed the number of children where all three judges were in agreement; if no agreement was to be found between the judges their rating were included under 'disagreement'. In the combined group, under PA were all the children where at least two judges from each

Child's serial No..........   Date..........

(1) *Voice quality*

    Deep ....

    Breathy ....

    Throaty ....

    Harsh ....

    Hoarse ....

    Strident ....

    Soft ....

    Nasal ....

    Fairly normal ....

    Normal ....

    Other ....

(2) *Pitch*

    Too high ....

    Too low ....

    Normal ....

    Other ....

(3) *Loudness*

    Too loud ....

    Too weak ....

    Normal ....

    Other ....

(4) *Intonation*

    Monotonous ....

    Irregular ....

    Some rise & fall ....

    Fairly normal ....

    Normal ....

    Other ....

(5) *Rate of speaking*

    Too rapid ....

    Too slow ....

    Jerky ....

    Monotonous ....

    Normal ....

    Other ....

FIGURE 4.1 Audit form for the recording and rating of speech.

group were in agreement and under FA were the children where all six judges were in agreement; all other cases were included under 'disagreement'. In the second study, as stated, there was only a single rating for each child and this is shown in the same table as the ratings of the partially-hearing children from the first study.

VOICE QUALITY

The ratings were as shown in Tables 4.1 and 4.2 The outstanding feature of these results concerning the voice quality of the deaf children

TABLE 4.1   Deaf children's voice quality

Voice quality	Panel of judges					
	Experienced		Inexperienced		Combined	
	PA	FA	PA	FA	PA	FA
Deep	4		1	2		
Breathy	5	5	2	3	1	1
Throaty	1	1		1		
Harsh	4	3	5	1	1	1
Hoarse	1					
Strident		3	1	2	1	2
Soft	2	1	1		1	
Nasal	1		2			
Fairly normal	5	2	4	4		
Normal	2		1			
Disagreement	18		28		50	

TABLE 4.2   Partially-hearing children's voice quality

Voice quality	Panel of judges						1980 study: Class teacher
	Experienced		Inexperienced		Combined		
	PA	FA	PA	FA	PA	FA	
Deep							
Breathy		2	2				1
Throaty			1				
Harsh							
Hoarse							
Strident							
Soft	1	1	2		1		
Nasal	1		3	1	1		2
Fairly normal	9	5	7	3	7	3	10
Normal	2	1					15
Disagreement	5		8		15		

was the considerable degree of disagreement in both panels of judges, disagreement being more pronounced among the inexperienced listeners. When the ratings of both groups of judges were combined agreement was almost negligible. Even so, note that nearly 16 per cent of the deaf children were rated by each panel of judges to have normal or near normal voice quality. According to the ratings of the experienced listeners nearly 42 per cent of the children had breathy, harsh, deep or strident voice qualities. The same adjectives were chosen by the inexperienced listeners to describe the voice quality of nearly 25 per cent of the children.

In the partially-hearing group disagreement between the two panels of judges was again quite high. It is interesting to note, however, that both panels of judges thought that more than half of the children had fairly normal or normal voice quality. In the second study the great majority of the children (90%) were rated by their teachers as having fairly normal or normal voice qualities. This is a very interesting result and it will be discussed later on in this chapter.

PITCH

The ratings were as shown in Tables 4.3 and 4.4. Disagreement within panels of judges was relatively low, varying from 7 to 15 per cent of the children. When the judges' ratings were combined, however, disagreement was very high, reaching just over 62 per cent of both the deaf and the partially-hearing children. Although teachers and lay people separately rated a considerable number of children as having either 'too high' (25%, 15%) or 'normal' pitch (15%, 27%) it is clear from Table 4.3 that they felt the pitch of just over 35 per cent of the deaf children could only be included under the heading 'other'. When asked for further explanation they unanimously responded by describing a voice with inappropriate rise and fall variation in pitch.

In the partially-hearing group both experienced and inexperienced listeners separately rated the majority of the children (55%) as having 'normal' pitch. In the 1980 study the percentage of children rated with normal pitch was nearly 90 per cent.

TABLE 4.3   Deaf children's pitch

Pitch	Panel of judges					
	Experienced		Inexperienced		Combined	
	PA	FA	PA	FA	PA	FA
Too high	8	7	2	7	2	3
Too low	3	2	4			
Normal	5	4	10	6	3	3
Other	12	10	16	4	11	
Disagreement	7		9		36	

TABLE 4.4   Partially-hearing children's pitch

	Panel of judges						1980 study: Class teacher
	Experienced		Inexperienced		Combined		
Pitch	PA	FA	PA	FA	PA	FA	
Too high			1				1
Too low	2		2	1	1		
Normal	5	10	8	7	6	2	25
Other	4	3	5	1	1		2
Disagreement	3		2		17		

LOUDNESS

The ratings were as shown in Tables 4.5 and 4.6. The speech loudness of the majority of the deaf children as rated by their teachers came under the headings 'normal' and 'other'. The inexperienced listeners thought that most of the deaf children had either 'normal' or 'too loud' speech. Note, however, that a substantial number of children were rated by each panel to have 'too weak' speech loudness. Both panels of judges tended to agree on the deaf children whose speech loudness was rated as either 'normal' or 'too loud'. Disagreement, however, between the two panels of judges was again very high. The teachers were asked to elaborate on their categorisation of 'other' and most of them responded that they assigned this category to those children whose speech loudness varied from sentence to sentence in an inappropriate manner. This point will be discussed later on in this chapter.

In the partially-hearing group both panels of judges agreed that the majority of the children, nearly 60 per cent, had 'normal' speech loudness.

TABLE 4.5   Deaf children's loudness

	Panel of judges					
	Experienced		Inexperienced		Combined	
Loudness	PA	FA	PA	FA	PA	FA
Too loud	3	4	7	6	3	3
Too weak	3	5	5		3	
Normal	7	6	16	9	8	4
Other	13	8	4		3	
Disagreement	9		11		34	

TABLE 4.6   Partially-hearing children's loudness

	Panel of judges						
	Experienced		Inexperienced		Combined		1980 study: Class teacher
Loudness	PA	FA	PA	FA	PA	FA	
Too loud			1	1			1
Too weak		2	1	2		2	1
Normal	4	17	9	9	10	6	26
Other		1		1			
Disagreement	3		3		9		

In the 1980 study the percentage of children with 'normal' speech loudness increased to nearly 93 per cent.

INTONATION

The ratings were as shown in Tables 4.7 and 4.8. Only very few of the deaf children were rated by either panel of judges to have 'fairly normal' or 'normal' intonation. The great majority of them were thought to have defective intonation patterns, either 'irregular', with 'some rise and fall' or 'monotonous'. When the ratings of both panels of judges were combined there was considerable agreement on the children whose intonation was judged to be either 'irregular' or with 'some rise and fall'. In all other cases disagreement was very high.

Among the partially-hearing children intonation ratings showed a slightly different picture, with more of them rated by each panel of judges

TABLE 4.7   Deaf children's intonation

	Panel of judges					
	Experienced		Inexperienced		Combined	
Intonation	PA	FA	PA	FA	PA	FA
Monotonous	5	4	4	1	2	
Irregular	15	4	13	4	10	
Some rise and fall	11	8	14	2	5	2
Fairly normal	1	1	4	1	1	1
Normal			1			
Disagreement	9		14		37	

TABLE 4.8   Partially-hearing children's intonation

	Panel of judges						1980 study: Class teacher
	Experienced		Inexperienced		Combined		
Intonation	PA	FA	PA	FA	PA	FA	
Monotonous	2		5		1		1
Irregular				1			
Some rise and fall	3		4	1	1		1
Fairly normal	4	1	3	1	2		2
Normal	4		2				24
Disagreement	13		10		23		

as having either 'normal' or 'fairly normal' intonation patterns. Disagreement between the two panels of judges was extremely high. In the 1980 study nearly 86 per cent of the children had normal intonation patterns.

RATE OF SPEAKING

The ratings were as shown in Tables 4.9 and 4.10. Both panels of judges rated the majority of the deaf children as having either 'too slow' or 'jerky' rate of speaking. Agreement between the two panels of judges on this was quite high. Note that only very few of the deaf children were judged to have 'normal' rate of speaking and none of them came under the category of 'too rapid' rate of speaking.

In the partially-hearing group both panels of judges gave the rate of speaking of just over half of the children as being either 'jerky' or

TABLE 4.9   Deaf children's rate of speaking

	Panel of judges					
	Experienced		Inexperienced		Combined	
Rate of speaking	PA	FA	PA	FA	PA	FA
Too rapid						
Too slow	12	2	8	6	7	
Jerky	15	10	18	9	18	1
Monotonous	5	3	2		1	
Normal	3	1	3	1	1	1
Disagreement	7		11		29	

TABLE 4.10 Partially-hearing children's rate of speaking

Rate of speaking	Experienced		Inexperienced		Combined		1980 study: Class teacher
	PA	FA	PA	FA	PA	FA	
Too rapid		1	1				
Too slow	2	1	2		2		6
Jerky	4	2	5	2	2		
Monotonous							
Normal	5	3	3	4	3	1	22
Disagreement	9		10		19		

'normal'. Agreement between the two panels of judges was low. In the 1980 study nearly 80 per cent of the children were considered to have 'normal' rate of speaking and the rest were rated as having 'too slow' rate of speaking.

SUMMARY

The most common errors affecting the prosodic or suprasegmental features of the speech of deaf children relate to intonation, phrasing, pausing, rate of speaking, breath control, stress, overall rhythm, loudness control, pitch control and, of course, voice quality. It is difficult to delineate each of these features and study their effects separately. They are intrinsically interwoven and thus any change, improvement or deterioration in any one of them is bound to affect the perception of the others. Having said this, however, the labels used provide a useful frame within which specific and important points can be made and discussed.

Intonation among deaf children is usually flat and monotonous or is characterised by irregular and inappropriate patterns of some rise and fall. Phrasing and pausing are usually inaccurate and tend to occur more frequently and at inappropriate locations. Breath control is defective, thus interrupting the natural flow of speech. Rate of speaking is generally slow and laboured, with wrong stress patterns and inappropriate emphasis. Speech loudness is often abnormal. In 1975 Calvert and Silverman suggested that the overall intensity of the speech of deaf children is generally reduced, which is certainly so for some deaf children but not for all. This is supported by the findings of Penn (1955) who reported that, of 1086 patients with marked sensorineural hearing losses, 'excessive volume' was a common vocal characteristic. The ratings presented previously also bear this out. Weak voices result primarily from inadequate use of the residual lung capacity and breathlessness whilst loud voices could result from an abnormally high respiratory driving force, excessive upper laryngeal resistance, or both. It is also documented that deaf children have limited control over their voice loudness. In one-to-one conversation, and in a relatively quiet room, deaf children's voices tend to be either normal or on the high side in terms of loudness. Great difficulties arise, however, when such children need to adjust the loudness of their voices to meet social and environmental constraints. For example, many deaf children find it extremely difficult to assess the acoustic or social environment in which they are functioning with the result that on the one hand they tend to speak loudly in places and circumstances requiring a quiet voice and on the other they fail to raise the loudness of their voice in order to alleviate some of the masking effects of competing background noise.

Pitch control is also defective. The pitch of a considerable number of deaf children is on the high side with inappropriate rise and fall variations. This, coupled with difficulty in loudness control, can create a very abnormal voice quality which is a formidable barrier to communication.

In addition to these errors and mainly because of them, many deaf children exhibit abnormal voice qualities which are detrimental to effective communication. The most common problems of voice quality encountered with deaf children include excessive breathiness, nasality, stridency and harshness.

The speech of partially-hearing children exhibited on the whole similar prosodic problems but to a far lesser degree and intensity than those exhibited by deaf children. The main reason for this is primarily the degree of hearing loss. There is no doubt that we learn to talk and later to control our speech mainly by auditory feedback. It is obvious then, that a hearing impairment will interfere partially or totally, depending on its severity, with this auto-corrective cyclical process. The severity of such interference is naturally less with partially-hearing children than with deaf children and this explains their better speech qualities.

Note, however, that the children in the 1980 study were on average deafer by 10 dB than the partially-hearing children included in the 1967 study. Yet the prosodic features of the speech of the 1980 children were more normal than those of the children in 1967. This discrepancy is probably due to the following reasons.

(a) The children in the 1980 study were using much better hearing aids than those used by the partially-hearing children in the 1967 study. In particular the hearing aids of the children in 1980 were giving a wide range of frequency amplification from 150 or 200 Hz up to

4000 Hz compared with the narrow range of frequency amplification (300 Hz to 3500 Hz) of the hearing aids used by the children in 1967. The wider range of frequencies amplified, especially at the lower end, is of crucial importance here, mainly because it is precisely these low frequencies that carry most of the hard core of prosodic information in speech.

(*b*) The children in the 1980 study were using binaural hearing aids as opposed to the monaural hearing aids used by the children in 1967. It is well known (Markides, 1977) that binaural hearing aids, because of the combined effects of binaural summation of energy, binaural summation of information and enhanced localisation, render amplified speech much more natural sounding, with depth and clarity, than monaural hearing aids.

(*c*) The assessors used in the 1980 study were the class teachers of the children. This was not so in the 1967 study.

CHAPTER FIVE

Speech intelligibility

This chapter is divided into three parts. The first part summarises the findings of recent studies dealing with the overall speech intelligibility of hearing-impaired children; the second part deals with relationships and prediction of speech intelligibility, and the third part presents and discusses the major factors affecting speech intelligibility.

RECENT STUDIES

The results obtained by Hudgins and Numbers (1942) and Sheridan (1948) with regard to speech intelligibility among deaf children have already been presented in Chapter 2 and they will not be restated here. Also, note that these two studies were carried out nearly four decades ago and their results may not reflect present-day conditions. The number of recent studies dealing formally with the speech intelligibility of deaf children is very small indeed. This is very surprising because the subject area is very important and relatively easy to investigate. Be that as it may, the relevant studies carried out on both sides of the Atlantic will now be described.

We start off with two reports from the Department of Education and Science (DES, 1964, 1972). Both of these reports provided brief details on the speech intelligibility of deaf children as assessed by a single listener. The first report gave information on the speech of 397 children whilst the second report dealt with the speech of 167 children. Speech intelligibility was rated on a three-point scale: intelligible, partly intelligible and unintelligible. The 1964 report stated that one-third of the children with hearing losses exceeding 80 dB HL in the better ear had speech which was unintelligible. The comparable figure for the 1972 report was 23 per cent. This discrepancy of 10 percentage points does not really reflect any improvement in speech intelligibility but most probably it is due to sampling variations.

Brannon (1964) studied the speech intelligibility of 20 hearing-impaired children drawn from a single day school. All the children were 12 to 15 years old and their individual mean hearing losses were in excess of 75 dB. He found that only 20 to 25 per cent of the words spoken by the children were intelligible to naive listeners, that is people without any previous experience with the speech of deaf children.

As stated, Markides' (1967) study involved 85 children: 58 deaf and 27 partially-hearing. All the children were drawn from two age groups, one group composed of 7-year-olds, the other of 9-year-olds. The hearing losses of the children were calculated by finding the average HL in dB in the better ear at the frequencies 500, 1000 and 2000 Hz. The children were divided into four categories on the basis of average hearing loss.

1 60 dB and below   ($N=20$)
2 61–80 dB   ($N=19$)
3 81–100 dB   ($N=24$)
4 101 dB and above ($N=22$)

The mean hearing loss of the deaf pupils was 95 dB HL whilst that of the partially-hearing was 57 dB HL. The speech intelligibility of the children was assessed in two ways.

The first procedure involved the recording of samples of spontaneous speech from the children. For this purpose each child was required to describe five unrelated pictures. The intelligibility of each child's speech was assessed by two panels of judges consisting of three persons each. The first group of judges was composed of trained teachers of the deaf. The second group of judges was totally naive with regard to speech of deaf children. The judges were not the same for all the children. Altogether 30 teachers of the deaf and 37 university students acted as judges. The speech intelligibility of each child was based on the average number of words understood correctly by each group of judges. These averages were expressed as a percentage of the total number of words produced by each child when describing all five pictures. Thus each child had two speech intelligibility scores, one from the teachers (experienced listeners) and one from the 'laymen' (inexperienced listeners).

The second procedure involved the same two panels of judges and their task was to rate the speech intelligibility of each child on a six-point scale:

1 Normal
2 Very easy to follow
3 Fairly easy to follow
4 Rather difficult to follow
5 Very difficult to follow
6 Unintelligible.

The results obtained with the first procedure were as follows:

(a) The total number of words in the recorded speech of the 58 deaf children was 825. On average the teachers or experienced listeners were able to understand correctly 254 of these words or nearly 31 per cent. The inexperienced listeners on average scored 160 words correct or just over 19 per cent. The comparable figures for the partially-hearing children were 563 words out of a total of 678 words correctly understood by the teachers (83%) and 516 words (76%) correctly understood by the 'lay' people.

(b) These figures show that the teachers who were experienced listeners, as expected, scored higher than the inexperienced judges. There was, however, a very high correlation ($r=0.94$) between the scores of the teachers and the laymen.

(c) As expected the speech intelligibility scores of the partially-hearing children were significantly higher ($p=0.01$) than those of the deaf children.

(d) In the deaf group the speech intelligibility of the older children was slightly better than that of the younger children, whilst in the partially-hearing group the situation was exactly the reverse. None of the mean differences obtained proved to be statistically significant.

(e) The speech intelligibility of the deaf children attending the different schools was more or less the same except in one school where the speech intelligibility of the children was significantly better.

(f) The intelligibility scores of the children decreased as hearing loss increased. The differences between the mean scores of the children in the various hearing loss categories were found to be statistically significant ($p=0.01$) except in the last case, i.e. when hearing loss categories 3 and 4 were compared, when no significant difference was found. The product-moment correlation coefficient between the intelligibility scores of the children and their respective average hearing losses in the better ear (averaged across 500, 1000 and 2000 Hz) was -0.71 ($r=-0.75$ between laymen's scores and hearing loss).

(g) The speech intelligibility of those children who were making good use of their individual hearing aids (as assessed by their teachers) was significantly better than the speech intelligibility of children who were not using their hearing aids properly and efficiently.

(h) The speech intelligibility of the hearing-impaired children who had some preschool training was slightly but not significantly better than that of the children who had not received such training.

(i) The speech of the hearing-impaired children coming from families of higher socio-economic status was slightly more intelligible than that of the children from the lower socio-economic strata.

(*j*) The speech intelligibility of the hearing-impaired children with higher intelligence (as rated by their teachers) was slightly but not significantly better than that of the hearing-impaired children with lower intelligence.

The second procedure involved the rating of the speech intelligibility of the children on a six-point scale. The results obtained showed a very high agreement between the judges. Their ratings, together with the corresponding speech intelligibility scores of the children are shown in Table 5.1. As expected the results showed that the inexperienced listeners found more difficulty in following the speech of the hearing-impaired children than did the teachers. It is interesting to note that even when half of the words spoken were understood correctly, speech was judged to be 'rather difficult to follow'. Note that the teachers found the speech of nearly 59 per cent of the children either very difficult to follow or unintelligible. The comparable figure for the inexperienced listeners was nearly 64 per cent.

Ling (1976) quoted two studies that dealt with the speech intelligibility of deaf children. The first study by Heidinger (1972) dealt with 20 children drawn from a residential school for the deaf. They were 10–14 years old and their hearing loss in the better ear was in excess of 85 dB. The three judges involved, all experienced teachers of the deaf, rated only 20 per cent of the children's words in short sentences as intelligible. Similar results were reported in the second study quoted (Smith, 1975). In this study 40 children in the age groups 8–10 and 13–15 years were included. They all exhibited hearing losses in excess of 80 dB at 1000 Hz in the better ear. Their word intelligibility was on average 18·7 per cent.

Between 1973 and 1975, Levitt and his associates (1976) carried out a longitudinal study of the communication skills of deaf children. They selected just over one hundred 10-year-old deaf children from 10 schools

TABLE 5.1   Ratings and speech intelligibility score

Speech intelligibility	Experienced listeners Intelligibility score %			Inexperienced listeners Intelligibility score %		
	N	Mean	Range	*N*	Mean	Range
Normal	1	100				
Very easy	15	94·7	100–84	6	92·8	100–84
Fairly easy	8	80·8	90–72	16	79·3	100–53
Rather difficult	11	53·2	79–23	9	48·3	72–14
Very difficult	19	32·0	52–10	21	19·9	45–0
Unintelligible	31	7·5	42·0	33	3·3	21·0

and they repeatedly assessed their communication skills over a three-year period. For speech intelligibility each child was required to describe two or more picture sequences. The speech samples elicited were tape recorded and later on they were rated by three listeners all of them familiar with the speech of deaf children. They found that on each assessment more than 70 per cent of the children were rated difficult or impossible to understand.

A large-scale investigation into the speech intelligibility of deaf children was carried out in 1978 by Jensema, Karchmer and Trybus. The results of this study were widely publicised and appeared in several papers such as Jensema and Trybus (1978); Karchmer and Trybus (1977); Karchmer, Trybus and Paquin (1978) and Trybus (1980). Their data were obtained from the classroom teachers of 978 hearing-impaired children in special education programmes throughout the United States. The teachers were asked to rate the speech intelligibility of the children as it would appear to a member of the general public. A five-point scale was used as follows:

1 Very intelligible
2 Intelligible
3 Barely intelligible
4 Not intelligible
5 Would not attempt to use speech.

Their results showed a significant relationship between degree of hearing loss and speech intelligibility. The correlation between hearing levels in the better ear and speech intelligibility ratings was -0.68. The proportion of children rated intelligible or very intelligible ranged from 90 per cent for those children with mean hearing losses of 55 dB or less in the better ear, down to 23 per cent for those children with a hearing loss in excess of 90 dB in the better ear.

By far the most extensive British study on the speech intelligibility of deaf children was reported by Conrad (1979). His data came from 468 prelingually deafened children (15–16$\frac{1}{2}$ years old) drawn from both schools for the deaf and units for partially-hearing children. He divided the children into the following five dB bands based on the average hearing level (250–4000 Hz) in the better ear of each child:

1 Up to 65 dB
2 66–85 dB
3 86–95 dB
4 96–105 dB
5 106 dB and above.

Two procedures were used in the assessment of the speech intelligibility of each child. The first procedure involved the headmaster of each school who was required to rate the speech intelligibility of each child (ratings to be made with inexperienced listeners in mind) on a five-point scale:

1 Wholly intelligible
2 Fairly easy to understand
3 About half understood
4 Very hard to understand
5 Effectively unintelligible.

The second procedure involved a formal test of speech intelligibility. Each child was required to read 10 sentences. The speech of each child was tape recorded and later on it was presented to a panel of inexperienced listeners (four to six assessors in each panel). Each assessor was given a copy of the sentences being spoken and his or her task was to listen carefully and insert two missing words, or two target words, in each sentence.

Generally speaking Conrad's results were in line with the findings of previous studies. He found a strong relationship between hearing loss and speech intelligibility. As hearing loss increased there was a steady decline in the proportion of children with reasonable speech. In the special schools 48 per cent of the children were considered to have speech that was either very hard to understand or effectively unintelligible. Nearly 74 per cent of the children with hearing levels in excess of 90 dB had speech that was practically unintelligible.

Recently Geffner and Freeman (1980) reported both on the articulatory and on the overall speech intelligibility of sixty-seven 6-year-old deaf children (average hearing level in the better ear 104 dB re ANSI). With regard to articulatory errors some of their findings have already been presented and generally speaking they were similar to those previously reported by Hudgins and Numbers (1942) and Markides (1967). The overall speech intelligibility of the children was very poor with 76 per cent of them having speech that was barely intelligible.

SUMMARY

The results presented, especially those relating to children with hearing losses in excess of 90 dB, paint a very gloomy picture and there can be no escape from the conclusion that the speech of the large majority of these children is unintelligible to the man in the street.

Many workers have attempted to explain this disappointing level of achievement in speech intelligibility by looking at the individual or combined effects of a number of major factors such as the pathology of deafness, its degree and causation, use of amplification, schooling and methods of instruction. Some of these factors will be presented and discussed later on in this chapter. Meanwhile it is pertinent to note that most of the children included in the American studies were primarily drawn from educational establishments following either a combined or a manual method of instruction. The deaf children in the British studies came from special schools, the majority of which profess to follow the oral method of instruction. The danger exists that the uninitiated may assume that what is professed is really taking place. Far from it. The large majority of the schools for the deaf in the United Kingdom follow what can be loosely referred to as combined methods of instruction with a considerable number of them being more manual than oral.

RELATIONSHIPS AND PREDICTION

RELATIONSHIPS

It has already been stated that in the 1967 study the present writer analysed the articulatory errors of the children and also assessed their speech intelligibility. The relationship between the various categories and types of articulatory errors and speech intelligibility scores are shown in Table 5.2. Since the product-moment coefficient of correlation may be thought of essentially as that ratio that expresses the extent to which changes in one variable are accompanied by – or are dependent upon – changes in a second variable, it is possible to use this ratio as a criterion of the relative importance of the different types and categories of articulatory errors in the speech intelligibility of the children.

The negative correlations between the articulatory errors and the speech intelligibility scores mean that as the frequency of errors increased the intelligibility scores decreased. The three highest ranking articulatory

TABLE 5.2   Correlation coefficients. Articulatory errors / Speech intelligibility

Categories and types of articulatory errors	Speech intelligibility	
	Teachers' scores	Laymen's scores
Error categories		
1 Vowel and diphthong errors	−0·68	−0·66
2 Initial consonant errors	−0·86	−0·87
3 Final consonant errors	−0·87	−0·87
4 Total consonant errors	−0·88	−0·87
Type of error		
5 Omissions (consonant errors)	−0·75	−0·76
6 Substitutions (consonant errors)	−0·40	−0·40
7 Distortions (consonant errors)	−0·08	−0·08
8 Total articulatory errors	−0·89	−0·87

error categories affecting speech intelligibility were categories 8 (total consonant, vowel and diphthong errors), 4 (total consonant errors) and 3 (final consonant errors). Among the types of error, consonant omissions showed the highest negative correlation with the speech intelligibility scores. The above findings show that consonants were more important than vowels for intelligibility and that both consonant and vowel errors gave the best predicted value of intelligibility.

The correlation coefficients obtained are in line with those previously reported by Brannon (1966) and later on confirmed by Smith (1975). It has been observed, however, that children with about the same number of segmental errors can exhibit widely different degrees of speech intelligibility (Smith, 1975). Most probably these differences are due to the influence of suprasegmental aspects of speech.

There is no doubt that there is a direct relationship between the suprasegmental or prosodic aspect of speech and speech intelligibility (Hudgins and Numbers, 1942; John and Howarth, 1965; Levitt and his associates, 1974). Experimental attempts to quantify this relationship, however, have been on the whole unsuccessful.

In the 1967 study the linguistic abilities of the children involved were also assessed in terms of use of language, speech comprehension and vocabulary. The correlation coefficients between the linguistic test scores and the speech intelligibility scores are shown in Table 5.3.

The scores of the children in the linguistic tests, especially in the first two tests, were highly positively correlated with their speech intelligibility scores. In other words, this shows that those children who did well in the linguistic tests also tended to have more intelligible speech. The same finding was later on reported by John and his associates (1976). This point will be discussed later on in this chapter.

PREDICTION

Very few studies have dealt with the prediction of speech intelligibility. Those that have attempted to do so have concentrated solely on the predictive power of the audiogram in relation to speech intelligibility.

TABLE 5.3   Correlation coefficients. Linguistic tests / Speech intelligibility test

Test	Intelligibility test	
	Teachers' scores	Laymen's scores
Use of language	$r=0.85$	$r=0.84$
Speech comprehension	$r=0.84$	$r=0.83$
Vocabulary	$r=0.55$	$r=0.56$

Markides (1967) reported correlations of -0.71 and -0.75 between degree of hearing loss and speech intelligibility. Similar correlation values were recently reported by Trybus (1980). Kyle (1977) stated that a simple mean of hearing loss at five frequencies (250–4000 Hz) provides the most reliable predictor of speech intelligibility.

The intelligibility scores of the children included in the 1967 study were plotted against their respective degrees of hearing levels in the better ear and the results are shown in Figure 5.1. The same figure also shows the intelligibility scores of the children falling within each one of the points of the rating scale used. The continuous lines encompass the intelligibility scores of nearly 90 per cent of the children whilst the dotted line traces the best fitting curve.

There are several important points arising from this graph. The relationship between degree of hearing loss and speech intelligibility is certainly there but this relationship is not as simple as the correlation of -0.71 implies. Children with similar hearing losses exhibit widely different speech intelligibility scores, especially those children with hearing losses in excess of 50 or 60 dB. This, of course, is a well known fact

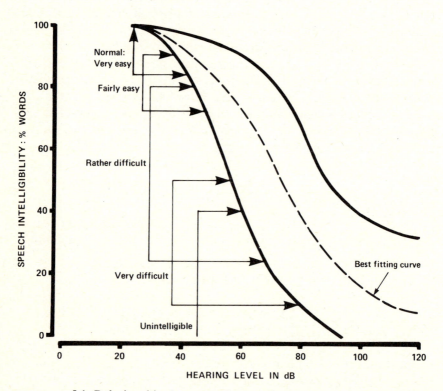

FIGURE 5.1 Relationship between degree of hearing loss and speech intelligibility

but it needs to be restated here so that the importance of the audiogram is put into its proper perspective.

Note also the wide range of intelligibility scores encompassed within each one of the points of the rating scale used. For example, the third point of the rating scale (rather difficult to follow) included children whose speech intelligibility scores varied from 24 per cent to 80 per cent. This enormous range may be partly due to such factors as voice quality, pitch, intonation, rate of speaking and rhythm.

Overall the results presented show that although there is an indisputable relationship between degree of hearing loss and speech intelligibility such a relationship must be interpreted with caution. Other factors such as age at onset of deafness and use of amplification, for example, are bound to affect this relationship.

In view of these uncertainties the writer initiated and is currently working on a project, the main aim of which is to assess the predictive value of the children's speech perceptual abilities on speech intelligibility. It hypothesised that the overall speech intelligibility of a prelingually deaf child depends not so much on the degree of hearing loss but on the child's ability to perceive and monitor speech through a combination of aided hearing and vision – the audio-visual perception of speech.

The results from a pilot experiment in this area show some interesting trends. Twenty-four prelingually deaf children varying in age from 9 years to 14 years took part. Their speech discrimination abilities were assessed separately under three modes of perception: the first mode involved only vision – lipreading; the second mode involved only audition – each child using his or her individual hearing aid(s); and the third mode was a combination of the first two – the audio-visual mode of perception of speech. The test used to assess the individual abilities of each child under each one of the above three modes was the video-taped Manchester Speechreading (Lipreading) Test (Markides, 1980*d*).

The speech intelligibility test involved each child describing 10 unrelated pictures with his or her responses being tape recorded and later on assessed by a number of inexperienced listeners who were required to write down on paper whatever they thought each individual child had said. The final intelligibility score of each child was based on the average number of words understood by the listeners expressed as a percentage of the total number of words produced by the child. The relationships between the speech discrimination abilities of the children and their respective speech intelligibility scores are shown in Figure 5.2.

Lipreading and speech intelligibility exhibit a positive but rather weak relationship ($r = 0.29$). The correlation between speech discrimination through audition and speech intelligibility is very high and of significant predictive power ($r = 0.87$). What is of enormous interest here, however, is the near linear relationship between the audio-visual perception of speech

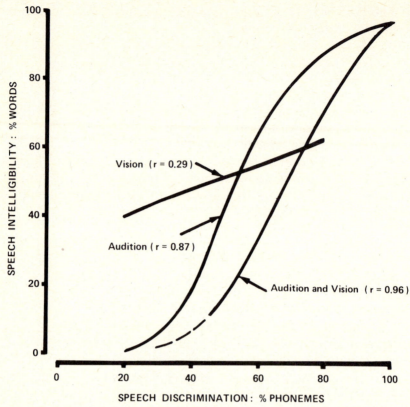

FIGURE 5.2 Relationship between speech discrimination abilities and
speech intelligibility

and speech intelligibility ($r = 0.96$). If this finding stands up to the rigours
of further experimentation we may in the future be able to predict the
speech intelligibility of prelingually deaf children with a high degree of
confidence.

SUMMARY

The degree of hearing loss in the better ear averaged across the main
speech frequencies (250–4000 Hz) has an undisputed predictive value
with regard to speech intelligibility. A better predictor of speech
intelligibility, however, seems to be the auditory speech discrimination
ability of the child and the best predictor so far suggested relates to the
audio-visual speech discrimination ability of the child. Further research is
recommended to verify or disprove this suggestion.

MAJOR FACTORS

There is a plethora of factors that can affect the speech intelligibility of deaf children. Some of these factors (voice quality, rhythm, misarticulations) have already been presented. Other major factors that need to be considered in some detail are the degree and type of hearing loss, use of residual hearing, educational environment, linguistic ability and, of course, speech teaching. This is by no means a comprehensive list of factors affecting the speech intelligibility of deaf children. Additional factors such as other handicap(s), intelligence, preschool guidance, calibre of teachers involved and the actual methodology employed in the teaching of speech can have considerable bearing on the speech of deaf children. Only the major factors will be discussed here.

PATHOLOGY OF DEAFNESS

It is generally accepted that the degree of hearing loss is one of the most important factors affecting the speech intelligibility of hearing-impaired children (Hudgins, 1934; Hudgins and Numbers, 1942; Sanders, 1961; Markides, 1967; Kyle, 1977). As hearing loss increases, articulation errors increase and overall speech intelligibility becomes worse. In 1962, however, Johnson in his study on the educational attainments and social adjustment of hearing-impaired children in ordinary schools, asserted that type of audiogram configuration rather than degree of hearing loss was the main factor affecting intelligibility. Johnson's assertion was later on refuted by Markides (1980a) who found that the speech intelligibility of three groups of children, representing three different pure tone audiogram configurations but with similar average hearing levels, were very similar. Time of onset of deafness is, of course, an obvious factor affecting speech intelligibility. It is true to say that a hearing impairment acquired later on in life affects speech intelligibility differently from a hearing impairment acquired at birth or very early in life. In the first instance, the individual affected has already learned the auditory cues for speech perception through normal auditory channels and in most cases such a disability can, to a large extent, be overcome by simply increasing the intensity of speech through the use of hearing aid amplification. In the latter case, however, the individual affected has to learn to speak through faulty auditory channels that receive, comparatively speaking, very little stimulation. As a result of this he may come to rely on different and fewer auditory clues for speech perception and this may well render him more susceptible to extraneous interference due to such things as noise, reverberation, change of speaker and change of hearing aid. In addition to these difficulties which arise either directly or indirectly from a hearing impairment, one must not overlook the possibility that whatever caused the hearing damage could also have caused further damage impinging on central processes in speech perception, i.e. integration and temporal sequencing problems, and difficulties in selective attention and short-term memory. These disorders are not easily detectable, especially when they are clouded by an obvious hearing impairment.

USE OF RESIDUAL HEARING

The provision of auditory experience for deaf children has been shown by Clark (1953), the Ewings (1957, 1958, 1964), and by many other workers to be important in furthering educational attainment. Markides (1967) found that the speech intelligibility of the deaf children who were making good use of their hearing aids was significantly superior to the speech intelligibility of the deaf children who were not. He also reported considerable differences between schools both in the amount of electronic amplification equipment available and in the efficiency with which such equipment was used. What is more disturbing, however, is the high incidence of misuse of individual hearing aids by children both in schools for the deaf and in units for the partially-hearing. The rate of misuse tends to increase with age and by the time the children leave school more than half of them do not make proper use of their hearing aid(s) (Markides, in preparation *a*). An important factor that interferes with the proper use of amplification in schools relates to the prevailing conditions. A considerable number of special schools for the deaf in the United Kingdom have inherited accommodation and environmental conditions that are not satisfactory for the proper functioning of hearing aids (John, 1957; Watson, 1964). What is even more depressing, however, is the fact that a considerable number of modern educational establishments for hearing-impaired children, especially units for partially-hearing children attached to ordinary schools, have been sited and designed without proper consideration pertaining to their acoustic environment, thus limiting the potential use of hearing aids.

EDUCATIONAL ENVIRONMENT

Markides (1967) reported significant variations between the speech intelligibility of deaf children attending different schools. This ties in well with the results obtained by Murphy (1957), Wollman (1961) and Redgate (1964) with regard to educational attainments. It is generally accepted that educational environment affects achievement especially in the case of handicapped children. Deaf children, for instance, because of their auditory handicap, are denied much of the incidental learning available to normal children both inside and outside the school. The special school has, therefore, to make good this deficiency and the degree of success in doing so depends mainly on the quality of education and the general ethos prevailing within the school. Many of the schools for the deaf, apart from being geographically isolated from each other, have long and well established traditions which might hinder communication of new ideas. Attitudes more suited to the nineteenth century possibly linger on and the setting of a low level of aspiration may well be one of the main reasons for low academic standards. Both Markides (1967) and John (1975) considered the educational environment and educational aspirations set by each school as one of the most important single factors affecting speech intelligibility, so much so that in many instances the degree and type of hearing loss become of secondary importance.

LINGUISTIC ABILITY

Both Markides (1967) and John (1975) reported a significant relationship between linguistic ability and speech intelligibility. Those children who performed better in the linguistic tests also tended to have better speech intelligibility. It may well be that a child who has a clear picture of what he wishes to say and who knows the correct method of putting words together will be able to speak more fluently, his rate of speaking will be more normal, and thus his speech intelligibility will be better. Ignorance of the correct meaning and use of language may cause a child to be uncertain and halting in his speech, thus speech intelligibility will suffer as a result of poor linguistic ability. On the other hand, a deaf child with good speech intelligibility, because of his ability to communicate to others in an understandable manner has an incentive to use his language and in the process of communicating he will naturally develop further his linguistic abilities.

SPEECH TEACHING

As far back as 1933 Haycock, commenting on the poor speech intelligibility of deaf children, attributed this mainly to 'inadequate and insufficient training and preparation to meet a continually growing and expanding set of varied speech requirements'. Hudgins and Numbers (1942) also thought that the speech intelligibility of deaf children was dependent on such factors as amount of time spent on speech training and the extent to which the habit of speech was cultivated. It was not surprising, therefore, to find (Markides, 1967) that the speech intelligibility of deaf children who were receiving systematic and consistent tuition on speech was significantly better than that of similar children who were not receiving such training. In the 1967 study only one school (of five schools visited) was providing individual and systematic speech teaching to the children. In all other cases no formal individual or class lessons on speech improvement were provided and any speech teaching that occurred was done incidentally and without any cohesive school policy. This was not a desirable situation. Unfortunately, however, speech teaching to hearing-impaired children in the last fifteen years has deteriorated even further. For example, in the last five years the present author came to know quite well 14 schools for the deaf and more than 30 units for partially-hearing children. Only in two of these schools was speech teaching carried out on an individual basis. None of the units was providing systematic speech training to the children. Surely this is an area for improvement?

SUMMARY

There is a plethora of factors affecting the speech intelligibility of hearing-impaired children. The most important are the ethos, speech environment and aspirations characterising the educational establishment, the pathology of deafness (especially its severity), the use of residual hearing and competent and consistent speech teaching.

CHAPTER SIX

Speech assessment

Black (1971) stated that 'the speech of deaf children differs from normal speech in all regards'. This all-embracing statement is certainly correct and the results of the numerous studies so far cited attest to this. Most of the faults occurring in the speech of deaf children have been adequately described but as yet we do not really know how they are interconnected. It is this lack of knowledge that makes the evaluation of deaf children's speech such a difficult task. The problem was well appreciated by Smith (1980) when she stated:

> The problem of evaluating the deaf child's speech is that the deaf child does not have one speech problem. The speech problems exist in bunches or, more accurately, in stacks. A bunch has the possibility of being taken apart so that one part can be tidied up at a time. A stack has one error built on another in some unknown order. This order may differ from one child to another, but each error is fastened to another. The complexity and interrelatedness of speech errors make evaluations extremely difficult.

Despite the difficulties involved evaluation must be carried out because without it the danger exists that speech remediation programmes will be based on incorrect premises. So far evaluative procedures have concentrated on the assessment of three major areas of speech: articulation, prosodic features, and overall speech intelligibility. The purpose of this chapter is to present and discuss the tests available and the assessment procedures involved in the evaluation of each one of these major components of speech.

ASSESSING ARTICULATION OR SEGMENTAL PRODUCTION

There are many articulation tests available. These include the Photo

Articulation Test (Pendergast, Dickey, Selmar and Sodir, 1969), the Edinburgh Articulation Test (Bogle and Ingram, 1971), the Goldman–Fristoe Test of Articulation (Goldman and Fristoe, 1972), the Ohio Test of Articulation and Perception of Sounds (Irwin, 1974), Ling's Phonetic and Phonologic Level Speech Evaluation (Ling, 1976), and the Templin–Darley Test of Articulation (Templin and Darley, 1969). Most of these tests originated in the USA and, apart from Ling's tests, they were all primarily designed and constructed to meet the needs of normal hearing children. A comprehensive list of these tests together with some pertinent comments on their suitability of use can be found in the paper by Levitt (1980). It needs to be stated here, however, that most of these tests usually examine a very extensive list of sounds in words or sentences which are beyond the linguistic competence of most deaf children. Also their administration and scoring is so time consuming and 'sophisticated' that both teachers and children find them frustrating and of limited use (Smith, 1980).

The linguistic composition of most of these tests is culture-bound and this makes them unsuitable for use with British children. In view of these difficulties the present author, in 1967 and again in 1980, constructed his own articulation tests, one of which is shown in Appendix 1. The tests are very simple in construction and straightforward in administration. They consist of a number of monosyllables, specially selected to be within the vocabulary abilities of the children, and test a representative number of the phonemes in the English language. Each word is represented pictorially and the child responds to each picture separately, his responses either being immediately transcribed phonetically by the teacher or tape recorded for assessment at leisure later on. Misarticulations are noted, categorised and quantified. The whole procedure is quick and within the abilities and resources of most class teachers of the deaf. This type of articulation test, however, has its disadvantages. It does not cover all English phonemes and their combinations, neither does it provide information regarding coarticulation abilities in sentences or running speech. Some workers have suggested the use of sentences or continuous discourse or both for testing articulatory proficiencies. This proposition, however, has not yet been accepted, mainly because the basic procedure is difficult to standardise and involves some degree of reading – a linguistic activity that can easily contaminate articulatory performance. Also continuous discourse increases the difficulty of phonetic transcription, thus making articulation testing too difficult for most teachers of the deaf.

The tests so far mentioned assess articulation at the phonetic level; they do not provide the teacher with information regarding the child's basic competence to articulate speech in a linguistic context. In other words most of the relevant tests available do not look at those articulatory abilities of a child which have already developed and form an integral part of his spontaneous language – his phonology. Periodic assessment of articulatory ability at the phonological level can provide substantial information on the child's speech progress.

The assessment procedures proposed by Ling (1976) are most suitable for this purpose. His phonetic and phonologic level speech skills evaluations have become very popular since their appearance. Basic articulation abilities are assessed at the phonetic level. At the phonologic level these skills are evaluated in the context of spontaneous speech. Ling's evaluation methods are very clear and very effective but require considerable expertise for proper administration.

ASSESSING PROSODIC OR SUPRASEGMENTAL PRODUCTION

There are very few tests that have been specifically designed to examine the prosodic or suprasegmental features of the speech of deaf children. One of these tests is the Preschool Connected Speech Inventory (DiJonson, 1971) which was designed to evaluate intonation and speech intelligibility in connected speech. It contains phrases and short sentences with picture clues. Its scope is very narrow and because of this it has not been widely used.

In 1976, Levitt and his associates developed the Prosodic Feature Production Test and used it in their longitudinal study. With this test they examined the ability of deaf children to produce three basic prosodic features: contrasting stress, intonation, and pause or juncture. The test contains six sentences varying in length from two to five syllables as shown in Figure 6.1.

The feature of stress is indicated by capital letters and underlining, pause by three dots, and intonation by a question mark. After adequate practice the child is asked to read the sentences, his responses being

---

Come here
Oh boy
He has one big dog
I want to see it
My new hat is blue

Methodological representation:
Come ... here   (pause)
COME here   (stress)
Come HERE   (stress)
Come here?   (intonation)

FIGURE 6.1 The Prosodic Feature Production Test

recorded for assessment later on by a panel of experienced listeners. This test sounds simple and straightforward but it is rather complicated and time consuming. Care needs to be taken so that the act of reading does not interfere with the fluency of speech production.

Other authors, including Ewing and Ewing (1964) and Markides (1967) used special rating scales to assess prosodic features such as voice quality, pitch, loudness, intonation and rate of speaking. This procedure involves the tape recording of representative samples of the child's spontaneous speech for assessment by a panel of listeners. Again, this procedure is time consuming and unless the listeners are experienced the ratings can be highly unreliable.

INSTRUMENTAL PROCEDURES

Nowadays instrumental procedures in the evaluation of speech are extremely sensitive and they can provide valuable and direct information on many physiological parameters of speech. For example, respiratory function during speech can be reliably and accurately measured by using respirometric techniques similar to those employed by Hixon, Saxman and McQueen (1967). Voice patterns including the determination of fundamental frequency (F_0) and the assessment of pitch changes can be reliably measured using oscillographic recordings and sound spectrography. Hypo- and hypernasality can be measured by using instruments such as the TONAR II. The laryngograph gives valuable information on pitch, intonation and stress and only a simple sound level meter is required to assess the intensity of speech.

The most widely used instrumental procedure in the assessment of speech is sound spectrography and in view of this more detailed discussion is warranted. Spectrographic analysis gives valuable information on four basic physical dimensions of speech (see Figure 6.2): (a) durational (horizontal axis of the graph), (b) frequency composition (vertical axis of the graph), (c) relative intensity of main frequency bands (variations of blackness of markings) and (d) vocal cord activity or fundamental frequency (pitch) of the voice. These four physical properties of speech convey valuable information relating to the voice and articulation of the speaker. In other words spectrographic analysis can give accurate information on the following: accuracy and distinctiveness of articulatory movements, absolute and relative duration of phonemes, the effect of adjacent sounds on articulation, differentiation between voiced and unvoiced phonemes, differences in frequency composition of phonemes, pitch control and its variations, intensity control, duration control of the prosodic aspect of speech, intonation and stress, and voice quality. Consider the specimens of spectrographic analysis: Figures 6.2 to

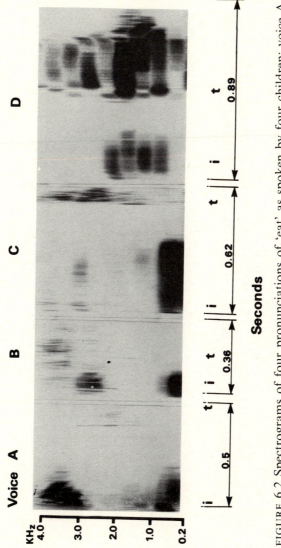

FIGURE 6.2 Spectrograms of four pronunciations of 'eat' as spoken by four children: voice A, normal hearing girl of 10 years; voice B, deaf boy of 10 years; voice C, deaf girl of 10 years; and voice D, deaf girl of 11 years

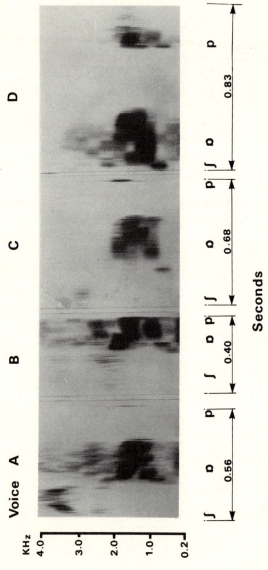

FIGURE 6.3 Spectrograms of four pronunciations of 'shop' as spoken by four children: voice A, normal hearing girl of 10 years; voice B, deaf boy of 10 years; voice C, deaf girl of 10 years; and voice D, deaf girl of 11 years

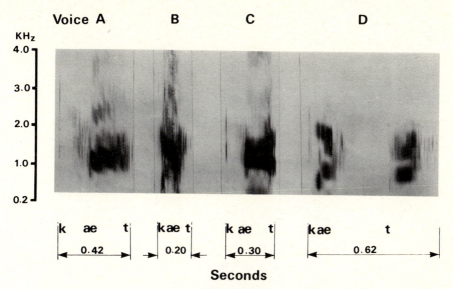

Voice A   B   C   D

FIGURE 6.4 Spectrograms of four pronunciations of 'cat' as spoken by four children: voice A, normal hearing girl of 10 years; voice B, deaf boy of 10 years; voice C, deaf girl of 10 years; and voice D, deaf girl of 11 years

6.5 are illustrations of spectrograms of four words spoken by one normally hearing girl and three hearing-impaired children. The four words analysed are 'eat' [it], 'shop' [ʃɒp], 'cat' [kæt], and 'knife' [naɪf]. Child A was a girl of 10 years with normal hearing, child B a deaf boy of 10 years, child C a deaf girl of 10 years, and child D was a deaf girl of 11 years.

Consider the word 'eat' spoken by the normally hearing girl (voice A). The vertical axis of Figure 6.2 represents linearly the frequency range from 200 Hz to 4000 Hz. The darkness of the trace indicates the relative energy level of the spectral components. For the vowel /i/ these frequency bands of concentrated energy or formants are expected to be at 250–400 Hz (first formant) and 2000–3300 Hz (second formant). There is additional scattered energy that contributes to a particular voice quality, provided of course such acoustic energy does not override or mask the basic characteristic formants of the vowel. Voice A has prominent concentrations of energy at the expected frequencies. The duration of the vowel /i/ is approximately 0·2 seconds followed by a period of silence of similar duration. This corresponds to the time the tip of the tongue blocked the outgoing air pressure. The sudden release of pressure caused an explosion which trailed into scattered frequencies centring around 2000 Hz. A careful examination of these formant bands reveals that they are made up of a number of discrete vertical striations each of which represents one complete vibration of the vocal cords. It follows therefore

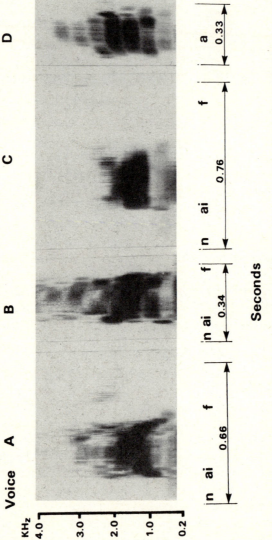

FIGURE 6.5 Spectrograms of four pronunciations of 'knife' as spoken by four children: voice A, normal hearing girl of 10 years; voice B, deaf boy of 10 years; voice C, deaf girl of 10 years; and voice D, deaf girl of 11 years

that the closer these striations are to one another the higher is the pitch of the voice. Overall the normally hearing girl took 0·5 seconds to produce the word 'eat'.

The spectrograms of voice B revealed some interesting characteristics. The vowels were comparatively short in duration and they were delivered in a loud staccato voice. No blockage of pressure was evident for the production of the final plosive consonants. In the word 'eat' the vowel /i/ was followed by random high frequency energy which was perceived as a distorted variation of /ʃ/. In the words 'shop' and 'cat' the final plosives were missing. In the word 'knife' there were slight traces of the initial nasal consonant /n/ but to all intents and purposes the final consonant /f/ was omitted.

The spectrograms of voice C had a lot of normal characteristics. The vowel /i/ in the word 'eat' was recognisable but slightly prolonged (0·36 seconds). There followed a period of silence which came to an end with a plosion for the pronunciation of /t/. The release of pressure introduced random energy throughout the frequency range which interfered with the crispness of the final /t/. The word 'shop' was intelligible. The initial consonant /ʃ/ was weak and the vowel /ɔ/ was slightly prolonged and neutralised. The final /p/ was produced in a crisp and perfectly normal manner. The word 'cat' was again intelligible although the final /t/ was omitted. The diphthong /aɪ/ in the word 'knife' was replaced by the neutral vowel /ə/ which was excessively prolonged. Both the initial nasal consonant /n/ and the final fricative consonant /f/ were rather weak. This girl spoke with a rising pitch, which appears in the figures as an increasing number of vertical striations per unit time in the temporal sequence of the vowels.

The spectrograms of voice D reflected many of the voice abnormalities of deaf speakers. The vowel /i/ in the word 'eat' was unrecognisable and was perceived as a very weak neutral vowel /ə/. The gap between the initial vowel /i/ and the release of pressure for the production of /t/ was there but following the release of pressure she introduced a very strong neutral vowel /ə/ followed by random energy around 1000 to 2000 Hz. The word 'eat' was perceived as two syllables [ətə́ʰ] with the stress on the second syllable. A similar observation can be made with the words 'shop' and 'cat'. Overall this girl took one and a half times longer to say the words than the normally hearing girl. The word 'knife' was totally unrecognisable. Both the initial and the final consonants were omitted and the diphthong /aɪ/ was produced as a strong variation of the neutral vowel /ə/. Note that this girl had difficulty in controlling the loudness of her speech. Some of her vowels were very weak whilst others were produced with excessive force. The analysis reflected speech that was monotonous – the fundamental frequency of her speech stayed the same and the formants of her vowels were predominantly straight.

ASSESSING OVERALL SPEECH INTELLIGIBILITY

Methods of assessing the speech intelligibility of deaf children basically involve the use of panel(s) of assessors. Their function is to listen to the speech of deaf children and either (a) write down whatever they think the child has said for later assessment leading to a percentage intelligibility score, or (b) rate the speech intelligibility of each child on a given scale, usually ranging from normal speech to unintelligible or no speech at all.

The assessment of speech intelligibility can be greatly affected by the way in which the speech material is elicited from the children, the mode of presentation of the children's speech, the relative sophistication of the assessors, and by the scoring procedures adopted.

SPEECH ELICITATION

The assessment of speech intelligibility necessitates the elicitation of representative samples, in sufficient quantity, of the children's speech. To achieve this one needs to take into consideration (a) the provision of favourable conditions and (b) the test materials and methods to be used.

It is important for the researcher to avoid generating tension among the children because this tends to influence their speech production adversely. One way to remove the stress inevitable in face-to-face testing is to record the samples of the children's speech. This procedure has been followed by most of the researchers in the field (Hudgins, 1934; Rawlings, 1936; Hudgins and Numbers, 1942; John and Howarth, 1965; Markides, 1967, 1980a).

With regard to the elicitation of speech from the children, two main methods have been followed in the past: the 'oral reading' method and 'picture description'. The oral reading method involved the reading aloud of lists of words (Hughson et al., 1941), phrases (Hudgins, 1934), or sentences (Voelker, 1935; Rawlings, 1936; Johnson, 1939; Hudgins and Numbers, 1942; Conrad, 1979). The picture description method was used by Sheridan (1948), Markides (1967, 1980a) and John et al. (1976).

Clark (1953), Davis and Silverman (1961), and Markides (1977) have criticised the oral reading method on the grounds that:

(a) oral reading does not represent speech in a social context;
(b) oral reading does not elicit representative samples of each child's speech;
(c) oral reading artificially manipulates the linguistic structure of the children's speech;
(d) oral reading interferes with the spontaneity of speech;
(e) oral reading puts a heavier burden on the children, especially those with reading difficulties;

(*f*) oral reading interferes with the temporal aspects of the speech of deaf children; and

(*g*) oral reading depresses the speech intelligibility scores of deaf children.

On the other hand, Kyle (1977) was of the opinion that picture description is not only a difficult and complex test of speech intelligibility but is also inaccurate. Conrad (1976) and Kyle and his associates (1978) favoured instead the oral reading method. Some of the reasons given in favour of the oral reading method were the following:

(*a*) it helps in 'practicalities of scoring which necessitate the identification of each attempted speech sound';

(*b*) it 'reliably reflects articulation rather than the mood of the child';

(*c*) it presents a simple task for the researcher and the listeners; and

(*d*) it can be easily standardised.

In view of this controversy, Markides (1978) compared the relative efficiency of the two methods. It was found that the speech intelligibility of the children elicited through picture description (mean intelligibility score 81·7%) was significantly superior ($p = 0·01$) to the intelligibility of their corresponding speech elicited through oral reading (mean intelligibility score 57·4%). It was concluded that picture description as opposed to oral reading provides a more realistic assessment of the speech intelligibility of hearing-impaired children.

When using pictures for elicitation of speech it is imperative to ensure that both the subject matter of each picture and the vocabulary required to describe each picture are within the abilities and interests of the children concerned. This method and the interview method, however, tend to interfere with the spontaneity of speech (albeit to a smaller degree than when reading lists of words, phrases or sentences) and also the speech samples elicited from each child when following these methods may be of widely different linguistic complexities. When using pictures it is necessary to employ several individual or groups of pictures or several picture sequences which need to be standardised, especially in terms of difficulty of description. The use of only one picture or picture sequence will almost inevitably interfere with the final assessment of speech intelligibility, mainly because of learning factors affecting the assessors. Davis and Silverman (1961) suggested that it would be helpful to capture the casual conversation of children for purposes of assessing speech intelligibility. In theory this is ideal; in practice it imposes formidable difficulties impinging on acceptable homogeneity of experimental procedures, and also it is a time-consuming undertaking.

MODE OF SPEECH PRESENTATION

Another important factor influencing the performance of the assessors is the mode of presentation of the speech to be assessed. Recently, Mineter (1982) carried out a small investigation in which she compared the speech intelligibility scores of 12 children achieved through an auditory and through an audio-visual approach. To start with each deaf child was video-taped whilst describing a series of unrelated pictures. For the auditory mode of assessment only the speech of the children was presented to the assessors. For the audio-visual mode of assessment the listeners were able both to hear and to see the child speaking (full face viewing on the monitor). It was found that the intelligibility of the speech of the children assessed by audio-visual means (mean intelligibility score 66·7%, standard deviation 18·95) was significantly superior ($p=0·01$) to the intelligibility of the same speech assessed by the auditory mode only (mean intelligibility score 53·5%, standard deviation 20·97). Individual differences varied from 3 to 24·1 percentage points with a group mean difference of 13·2 percentage points. Had the listeners also known of the subject matter being spoken about the differences would have been even greater.

ASSESSORS

Regarding the selection of listeners to assess the speech intelligibility of deaf children, it is noted that previous writers used either people familiar with the children's speech (teachers of the deaf – sophisticated listeners) or people to whom the speech of deaf children was completely strange (inexperienced or unsophisticated listeners) or both sophisticated and unsophisticated listeners. There is general agreement, however, that a realistic assessment of the speech intelligibility of deaf children must be based on the responses of unsophisticated listeners, mainly because teachers of the deaf, being accustomed to such speech, tend to overestimate its intelligibility (Markides, 1967).

The comparative ability of experienced and inexperienced listeners in assessing the speech intelligibility of deaf children have been systematically studied by a number of workers. Their results are summarised in Figure 6.6. They all agree that experienced listeners understand the speech of deaf children better than inexperienced listeners. In terms of intelligibility scores the differences obtained between the two groups of listeners varied from 5 to 25 percentage points.

For comparative purposes it seems essential to use the same group of listeners in evaluating speech intelligibility. This may not be a crucial factor affecting the results. Previous workers such as Hudgins and Numbers (1942), Clark (1953), John and Howarth (1965) and Markides

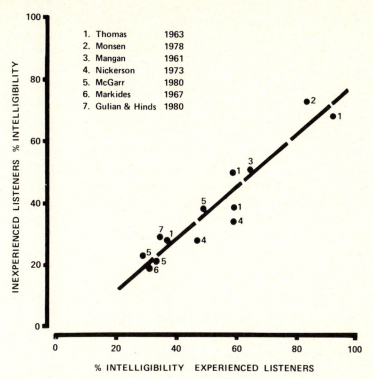

FIGURE 6.6 Relationship between intelligibility scores obtained by experienced and inexperienced listeners in studies on the speech of the deaf

(1967) have found little or no difference between the performances of
different assessors within a homogeneous group when assessing the
speech intelligibility of deaf children. Both Hudgins and Numbers and
Clark used as assessors a group of persons who had considerable
experience with deaf children. John and Howarth used instead groups of
lay people, while Markides used separately both groups of lay people and
groups of teachers of the deaf.

SCORING

Methods of scoring speech intelligibility tests show wide variations.
Johnson (1939) scored the speech intelligibility of deaf children by
awarding 10 points to sentences understood correctly the first time, 5
points to sentences understood correctly the second time and 2 points to
sentences understood correctly the third time. Hudgins and Numbers
(1942) scored speech intelligibility by awarding 10 points to sentences
fully understood – no points were given for partially correct interpretations. John and Howarth (1965) scored speech intelligibility in two ways:

first, on the number of words understood correctly; second, on the recognition of the complete syntactic pattern of the children's speech. Markides (1967, 1980*a*) scored speech intelligibility on the average number of words understood correctly by the assessors expressed as a percentage of the total number of words actually produced by each child. Conrad (1979) scored speech intelligibility on the mean number of 'target' words (two target words in each of 10 sentences read aloud by each child) correctly identified by a group of listeners.

It is clear that the method of scoring used by Johnson and by Hudgins and Numbers gave an underestimation of the children's speech intelligibility because no consideration was given to the partial successes of the children. Conrad's method of scoring was restrictive. It was based solely on two target words within a sentence to the exclusion of the intelligibility of the rest of the words comprising each sentence.

RATING SCALES

The assessment of the speech intelligibility of deaf children based on the number of words, phrases or sentences correctly understood by a panel of listeners is lengthy and time consuming and very few teachers of the deaf have the time or are willing to undertake such a task on a routine basis. A considerable number of teachers of the deaf and researchers in this area are instead using a rating procedure to obtain a quick assessment of overall intelligibility. There is no doubt that rating procedures can be highly unreliable. Provided, however, the rating scale used is logical and clear in its construction and wording and the assessors are experienced listeners who know exactly what they are doing, then rating procedures do represent a way of judging speech intelligibility without an inordinate investment in the listeners' time or a need for very expensive equipment. When large numbers of hearing-impaired children are involved the rating scale is the only practical way of assessing speech intelligibility.

The most widely used rating scales of speech intelligibility have already been mentioned in the previous chapter and there is no need to repeat them here. Suffice it to say that there are very few substantial differences between them and preference of one over the other is essentially personal.

SPEECH SCHEDULES

Mainly because of the lack of standardised tests and procedures in the assessment of the speech of hearing-impaired children individual attempts have been made to fill this gap by constructing and using speech schedules. The author came across several of these speech schedules in schools for the deaf and although their use is by no means widespread the teachers involved found them helpful and practicable. These schedules are used as a basis for assessing the intelligibility and structure of the speech of hearing-impaired children and they contain items such as voice quality, intonation, loudness, pitch, rate of speaking, speech comprehension, length of sentence, sentence structure, continuity of utterance, articulatory abilities and overall speech intelligibility. Obviously there are a lot of drawbacks in a non-standardised development schedule of assessment but periodical use made of it can provide reliable information to the teacher regarding the quality of speech and progress made by the children in her class. The Ewings (1964) made extensive use of such a procedure and their schedule is hereby reproduced although it needs to be noted that the present author finds its contents rather limited. The basic idea involved, however, is highly commendable and teachers of the deaf can easily improve on it to meet their own particular needs.

Schedule for assessing the intelligibility and structure of speech (Ewing and Ewing, 1964):

1 *Voice quality:*
   (*a*) deaf
      (i) abnormally high
      (ii) excessively laryngeal
   (*b*) fairly normal
   (*c*) near normal
   (*d*) normal.
2 *Intonation:*
   (*a*) monotonous phonation
   (*b*) some rise and fall of pitch
   (*c*) normal.
3 *Length of sentence.*
4 *Continuity of utterance:*
   (*a*) most words separately uttered
   (*b*) words sometimes joined together
   (*c*) words often joined together
   (*d*) words joined as in normal speech.
5 *Rate of speaking:*
   (*a*) drawled and laboured
   (*b*) slow with some rhythm
   (*c*) quick with some rhythm
   (*d*) quick and normally rhythmic.
6 *Sentence structure:*
   (*a*) word order often abnormal
   (*b*) word order normal but sentences incomplete
   (*c*) word order normal and grammar correct.
7 *Consonants correctly articulated*

SUMMARY

With regard to articulation it is reasonable to conclude that a simple test based on monosyllables and examining a representative number of the English phonemes plus Ling's phonological evaluation can be an acceptable and effective class and research procedure in the assessment of the articulatory abilities of deaf children. Assessment of the prosodic features of speech is a lengthy procedure involving panels of assessors. There are, of course, sophisticated ways involving expensive instrumentation which can provide additional information both on the articulatory and suprasegmental aspects of speech. Such procedures, however, are not easily accessible to the class teacher and because of their sophistication they may in fact impede rather than promote the desirability of carrying out periodic speech assessments.

It seems that the least objectionable method of assessing the overall speech intelligibility of deaf children entails:

(a) elicitation of representative samples of each child's speech in sufficient quantities, in excess of 40–50 words per child;

(b) the use of standardised groups of individual pictures or picture sequences or both, the content of which is within the experience of the children and the description of which is within the vocabulary abilities of the children;

(c) the recording of the children's responses;

(d) the use of groups of inexperienced listeners acting as assessors; and

(e) the scoring of speech intelligibility to be based on the average number of words understood correctly by the assessors expressed as a percentage of the total number of words produced by each child.

Generally speaking rating scales of overall speech intelligibility are less reliable than the percentage intelligible score method. They are quick to administer, however, and when the numbers of children involved are quite large they are the only practical way of assessing speech intelligibility.

Routine assessment of the speech of hearing-impaired children is an essential part of an ongoing speech teaching programme. At present speech assessment procedures are lengthy and time consuming and they are more relevant to the researcher than to the class teacher. There is a need to make them shorter and less sophisticated if they are going to be implemented with regularity in schools. In the absence of any formal and standardised tests for speech assessment the use of speech schedules is encouraged.

CHAPTER SEVEN

National survey on the speech intelligibility of hearing-impaired children

INTRODUCTION

In the autumn of 1981, the author circulated a letter to all schools for the deaf and to all units for partially-hearing children (PHUs) in England, Wales and Scotland inviting each class teacher to cooperate in a national survey on the speech intelligibility of hearing-impaired children. This survey also requested other relevant information on the pupils such as age, sex, residential status, cause of deafness, additional handicaps and degree of hearing loss. The main purpose of the survey was to find out what the class teachers themselves thought of the speech intelligibility of their pupils. The data were collected within a period of three months, from the end of October 1981 to the end of January 1982. They are presented here in broad outlines – detailed analysis and discussion will follow later on in educational and scientific journals.

PARTICIPATION

As stated a written request to participate was sent to each school for the deaf and to each PHU in England, Wales and Scotland. The list of these educational establishments and their addresses were obtained from the 1981 leaflet 'Educational provision for hearing-impaired children' issued by the National Deaf Children's Society.

UNITS FOR PARTIALLY-HEARING CHILDREN

These are special classes entirely of hearing-impaired pupils but located in ordinary schools where hearing children also attend. Although these educational facilities are referred to as PHUs a growing number of the children attending them are very deaf indeed.

Participation was requested from 449 PHUs. Of these, 24 were no longer functioning and 17 requests were returned marked 'Address not known'. The data submitted by 16 PHUs were not included in the final analysis – the data from 7 of these units were inadequate and 9 units submitted information too late for analysis. The number of PHUs participating was 272, which is nearly 70 per cent of all the units contacted in England, Wales and Scotland.

Information was submitted by 375 unit teachers and it covered 2429 pupils. Figure 7.1 shows more details on the pupil population of these units. Most of them were catering for 5 to 10 children each. A considerable number of them, however, were functioning with less than 4 children each. On the other hand a number of units were substantially bigger, in terms of pupil population, than several existing schools for the deaf. The average number of children in each unit was 8·9 and there is no indication at present whether this number will increase or decrease in the immediate future.

SCHOOLS FOR THE DEAF

Both day and residential schools for the deaf are included in this category. These schools are devoted primarily to the education of deaf children but as we shall see later on the pupil population of a considerable number of them is rapidly changing with a large number of their children having additional handicaps.

Participation was requested from 56 schools for the deaf but not all of them were able to cooperate. Information was received that 5 of them were no longer functioning and the data from 1 school were submitted too late for analysis. Only 1 school for the deaf refused to cooperate. Six schools did not respond to the request and the remaining 44 schools, or nearly 88 per cent of the schools for the deaf in England, Wales and Scotland submitted all information requested.

The submitted information covered 2743 pupils. The number of class teachers participating was 463. Figure 7.2 shows detailed information on the pupil population of the schools participating. The number of pupils in most schools for the deaf varied between 30 and 70. Note, however, that 6 of these schools were catering for less than 20 children each. In the next few years some of these schools may find it rather difficult to justify their existence. Eight schools had more than 100 children each but only one had more than 150 pupils. The average number of children in each school was 62·3.

PUPIL CHARACTERISTICS

This section presents the characteristics of the pupils with regard to age,

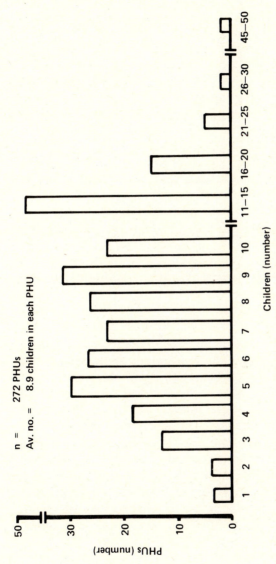

FIGURE 7.1 Distribution of hearing-impaired pupils in PHUs

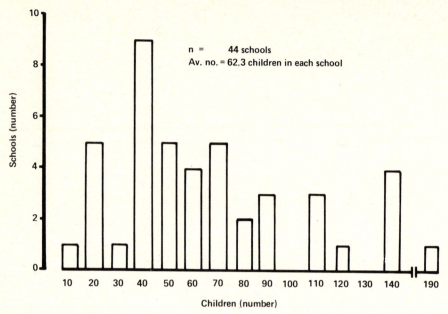

FIGURE 7.2 Distribution of hearing-impaired pupils in schools for the deaf

sex, residential status, cause of deafness, additional handicaps and degree of hearing loss.

AGE

Figure 7.3 shows the number of pupils in each age group from 2 to 19 years, attending the participating PHUs and schools for the deaf. The number of pupils in schools for the deaf showed a steady increase with increasing age reaching a peak at the 12 to 16 years age group and thereafter falling rapidly. The same pattern was observed with the number of children attending PHUs, although the variation in numbers of pupils from year to year was not as great as the one observed in schools for the deaf. The highest numbers of pupils in the PHUs were in the 10 to 14 years age groups. It is interesting to note that at present relatively more hearing-impaired children are channelled into PHUs rather than into schools for the deaf, and this tendency will certainly affect the future of a considerable number of schools for the deaf.

When the pupil populations of PHUs and schools for the deaf are seen together the most important point emerging is the rapid and steady decline in pupil numbers especially during the years from 1970 to 1977. During this period the number of hearing-impaired children attending these two educational facilities dropped by nearly 62 per cent. This drop can be partly explained by the falling birth rate (25% drop from 1970 to

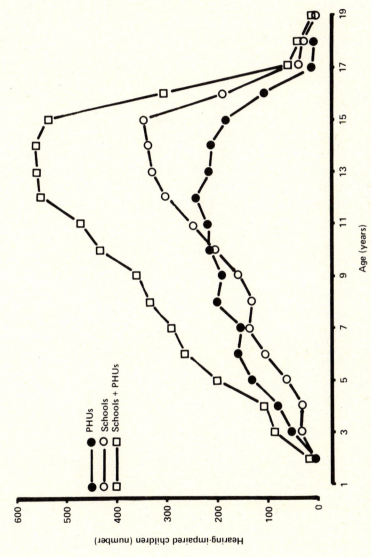

FIGURE 7.3 Distribution of hearing-impaired pupils by age in PHUs and schools for the deaf

1977), by the fact that more and more hearing-impaired children are educated in ordinary classes with the help of peripatetic teachers of the deaf, and also by the beneficial effects of preventive medicine and improved perinatal management.

If the same trend continues, within the next decade the number of hearing-impaired children attending schools for the deaf may decline further by as much as 40 to 50 per cent. Bear in mind, however, that at present the birth rate is actually rising and also that predictions of trends in birth rate are notoriously unreliable.

SEX

Table 7.1 shows separately the number and percentage of male and female pupils in each age group attending the PHUs and the schools for the deaf. There are slight variations from age group to age group regarding male/female composition but generally speaking just over 50 per cent of the pupils reported to this survey were males; this is virtually identical to what has been found in the United States (Karchmer, Milone

TABLE 7.1   Pupils' sex by age and educational facility

Age group in years	PHUs				Schools for the deaf			
	M	%	F	%	M	%	F	%
2	3	75·0	1	25·0	5	71·4	2	28·6
3	24	46·1	28	53·9	11	31·4	24	68·6
4	48	60·7	31	39·3	18	58·0	13	42·0
5	78	59·0	54	41·0	44	64·7	24	35·3
6	81	48·7	85	51·3	64	61·5	40	38·5
7	75	49·0	78	51·0	82	59·8	55	40·2
8	103	51·5	97	48·5	78	57·7	57	42·3
9	102	51·2	97	48·8	95	58·6	67	41·4
10	119	55·0	97	45·0	118	54·6	98	45·4
11	119	53·6	103	46·4	143	56·9	108	43·1
12	131	52·6	118	47·4	169	55·5	135	44·5
13	123	55·4	99	44·6	190	56·5	146	43·5
14	114	52·7	102	47·3	199	57·6	146	42·4
15	97	52·7	87	47·3	189	53·8	162	46·2
16	57	51·3	54	48·7	109	56·1	85	43·9
17	6	35·2	11	64·8	18	50·0	18	50·0
18	4	66·6	2	33·3	13	44·8	16	55·2
19	1				2	100·0		
Totals	**1285**	**52·9**	**1144**	**47·1**	**1547**	**56·3**	**1196**	**43·7**

and Wolk, 1979) and in Canada (Karchmer, Allen, Petersen and Quaynor, 1982).

RESIDENTIAL STATUS

The children attending the PHUs were all day pupils. Table 7.2 shows the residential status of the pupils in schools for the deaf according to age and sex. The same information is shown graphically in Figure 7.4. As expected most of the younger pupils were attending schools for the deaf on a day basis but with increasing age there was a steady increase in the number of boarders. Very few of these pupils were long-term boarders; most of them were weekly boarders. Overall just over 55 per cent of the pupils were boarders. There were slight variations in residential status according to sex with slightly more girls than boys being day pupils.

CAUSES OF DEAFNESS

It is acknowledged that the information on causes of deafness presented can be unreliable due to numerous sources of error, such as inaccuracy of

TABLE 7.2   Pupils' residential status by age and sex

Age group in years	Male %			Female %			Male & female %		
	N	D	B	N	D	B	N	D	B
2	5	100·0		2	100·0		7	100·0	
3	11	100·0		24	95·8	4·2	35	97·1	2·9
4	18	94·4	5·6	13	100·0		31	96·8	3·2
5	44	97·7	2·3	24	79·2	20·8	68	91·2	8·8
6	64	84·4	15·6	40	80·0	20·0	104	82·7	17·3
7	82	67·1	32·9	55	65·5	34·5	137	66·6	33·6
8	78	71·8	28·2	57	80·7	19·3	135	75·6	24·4
9	95	65·3	34·7	67	65·7	34·3	162	65·4	34·6
10	118	52·5	47·5	98	56·1	43·9	216	54·2	45·8
11	143	49·0	51·0	108	55·6	44·4	251	51·8	48·2
12	169	43·8	56·2	135	37·8	62·2	304	41·1	58·9
13	190	38·4	61·6	146	45·9	54·1	336	41·7	58·3
14	199	41·2	58·8	146	52·1	47·9	345	45·8	54·2
15	189	39·7	60·3	162	50·0	50·0	351	44·4	55·6
16	109	33·0	67·0	85	43·5	56·5	194	37·6	62·4
17	18	22·2	77·8	18	44·4	55·6	36	33·3	66·7
18	13		100·0	16	6·3	93·8	29	3·4	96·6
19	2		100·0				2		100·0
2–19	1547	50·4	49·6	1196	54·4	45·0	2743	56·4	43·6

D – day pupils
B – boarders

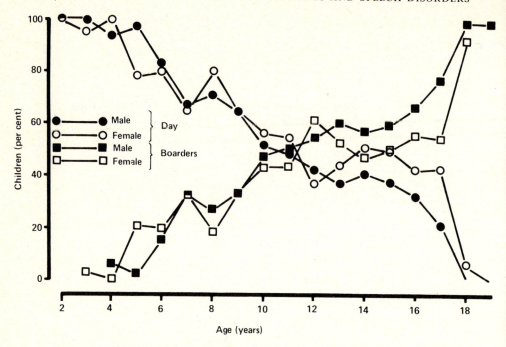

FIGURE 7.4 Residential status of hearing-impaired pupils in schools for the deaf shown by age and sex

diagnosis, incomplete school records and lack of medical evidence. The causes of deafness reported here were those known to the educational establishments participating in the survey and they must be treated as such.

Figure 7.5 shows the most common causes of deafness reported. More detailed information according to age is shown in Appendices 2 and 3. Cause of deafness in nearly 55 per cent of the pupils in PHUs and in nearly 47 per cent of the pupils in schools for the deaf was unknown. Maternal rubella accounted for 12·5 per cent of the children in PHUs and for 19·2 per cent of the children in schools for the deaf. The corresponding figures associated with heredity were 7·4 per cent and 6·7 per cent respectively. In all other cases, except for meningitis in schools for the deaf (6·7%), the figures reported were less than 5 per cent.

ADDITIONAL HANDICAPS

Overall, 16·3 per cent of the pupils in the PHUs and 20·9 per cent of the pupils in the schools for the deaf were reported by the class teachers to have one or more handicaps in addition to hearing loss. This percentage was relatively constant in PHUs but it varied widely among schools for

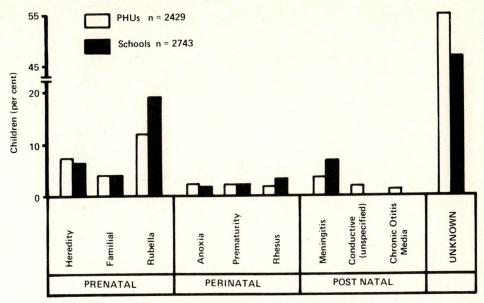

FIGURE 7.5 Most common causes of deafness

the deaf – some schools reported as low as 5 per cent and some as high as 90 per cent of their pupils having additional handicaps. Detailed information on additional handicaps by age is shown in Appendices 4 and 5. Figure 7.6 shows the most common additional handicaps reported. Note that mental retardation and visual problems were the most frequent additional handicaps quoted. Contrary to popular belief the number of pupils with behaviour, social and emotional problems (maladjustment) was very low; one pupil in a hundred.

DEGREE OF HEARING LOSS

The survey requested audiological information on each pupil in the form of unaided pure tone thresholds in the better ear at 250, 500, 1000, 2000 and 4000 Hz in dB ISO. As expected, for a number of children (1·1%) this information was not available, mainly because they were too young to cooperate in pure tone testing. No responses, in one or more frequencies, were reported in 4·7 per cent of the children – most of them from schools for the deaf. When calculating average hearing levels the 'No responses' were entered as 120 dB and those children without a pure tone audiogram were excluded.

It is accepted that the accuracy of the information supplied with regard to degree of hearing loss varied considerably from school to school depending on factors such as audiological facilities available, calibration

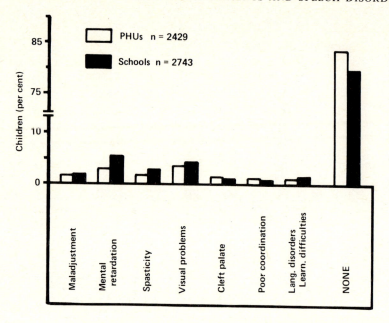

FIGURE 7.6 Most common additional handicaps

and maintenance of equipment used, and professional expertise. Had this been a small survey, in terms of numbers of pupils participating, the variations in accuracy would have contaminated the results considerably. However, in view of the large number of children involved any contamination of results is bound to be small and in this case it can be safely ignored.

The hearing levels reported were averaged by sex and by age group. It was found that the average hearing levels (AHL) of the boys and of the girls in each frequency (250 Hz to 4000 Hz) were virtually identical. This was true for both PHUs and schools for the deaf. In view of the similarity of the AHL among boys and girls the two sexes were combined and their AHL are shown by age, for PHUs in Table 7.3 and for schools for the deaf in Table 7.4. Similar information is shown graphically in Figure 7.7.

The AHL of the pupils in each age group were remarkably similar in terms of audiogram configuration. As expected the pupils attending PHUs had on average better hearing than those attending schools for the deaf. The differences observed were uniform varying from 18 to 25 dB (mean 22 dB) in each one of the main speech frequencies. This does not apply to age groups 2, 3, 18 and 19. The pupils involved in these age groups were either too young or too few or both to make any comparison worthwhile.

TABLE 7.3   Average hearing levels in dB (better ear): children in PHUs

Age groups in years	N	Frequency in Hz									
		250		500		1000		2000		4000	
		Mean	SD	Mean	SD	Mean	SD	Mean	SD	Mean	SD
2	2	85·0		88·7		97·5		97·5		102·5	
3	42	81·6	24·9	87·5	23·6	94·7	25·2	97·7	26·7	100·2	28·1
4	79	68·1	29·8	73·2	28·3	79·0	28·4	83·8	27·5	86·8	28·4
5	130	68·0	27·1	72·7	24·4	79·5	26·9	84·1	28·0	86·7	29·4
6	166	66·2	26·5	74·2	25·7	82·7	24·7	85·0	26·2	86·8	26·8
7	152	60·2	25·9	69·1	26·9	77·6	26·6	80·0	27·7	81·6	26·6
8	200	62·7	25·7	71·9	26·9	78·8	27·0	83·0	25·9	81·5	27·3
9	199	57·6	25·9	67·8	25·2	77·6	25·4	81·7	25·1	83·0	26·3
10	216	58·9	28·6	66·9	27·1	75·3	26·5	78·9	27·8	79·8	27·2
11	220	57·7	26·7	64·8	27·2	73·8	26·7	77·3	26·7	78·9	27·6
12	249	56·4	24·7	63·9	24·6	74·2	25·3	76·9	26·5	78·5	27·0
13	222	53·6	26·8	61·4	26·7	71·9	26·9	76·8	26·4	78·7	27·6
14	216	52·1	25·2	61·5	24·9	71·9	25·2	77·4	25·6	81·0	26·9
15	184	49·8	24·3	57·4	25·7	66·3	25·5	72·0	25·2	75·4	27·1
16	111	52·5	27·4	62·2	27·2	70·9	26·5	76·4	27·7	81·1	26·9
17	17	51·7	27·9	60·8	28·7	76·1	31·4	86·4	28·7	92·6	31·0
18	6	71·6	12·1	82·5	12·9	105·0	17·6	106·6	18·8	105·0	23·2
2–18	2411	58·5	27·0	66·6	26·6	75·5	26·6	79·6	26·9	81·5	27·5

The AHL quoted, must not be used to obscure the fact that a considerable number of children in PHUs were very deaf indeed. Note, for example, the high values of the standard deviations (SD) shown in Tables 7.3 and 7.4. In fact the AHL of the pupils (averaged across the frequencies 250 Hz to 4000 Hz, in the better ear) in PHUs have been constantly deteriorating with each consecutive age group since the early 1970s (Figure 7.8). To a certain extent the same can also be said for the pupils in schools for the deaf. In the latter case, however, the rate of increase in the severity of hearing loss has not been as great as that shown by the pupils in PHUs.

RATED SPEECH INTELLIGIBILITY

It needs to be emphasised again that the data reported here were obtained from the class teachers. Each teacher was requested to use her own extensive knowledge of the speech intelligibility of each child in her class and to rate it, as perceived by her, using the following seven-point scale.

TABLE 7.4   Average hearing levels in dB (better ear): children in schools for the deaf

Age groups in years	N	Frequency in Hz									
		250		500		1000		2000		4000	
		Mean	SD	Mean	SD	Mean	SD	Mean	SD	Mean	SD
2	3	92·1		97·8		97·1		98·5		105·0	
3	20	85·5	17·4	92·7	17·0	100·2	16·4	102·1	15·8	106·5	15·1
4	30	87·4	22·0	94·5	19·9	100·8	17·5	101·6	17·3	103·2	19·3
5	65	83·0	22·8	93·7	20·9	100·2	20·1	103·3	19·9	104·0	21·9
6	100	87·3	19·5	95·8	18·6	101·0	18·9	103·5	17·9	103·9	20·3
7	133	83·0	21·8	93·0	20·2	101·7	18·9	104·9	18·9	105·6	20·2
8	135	83·7	16·9	94·5	17·2	102·1	17·3	104·9	17·5	105·7	18·6
9	160	78·9	20·3	90·6	19·6	100·4	18·1	102·8	19·4	107·5	41·4
10	210	75·4	20·9	87·3	20·2	97·3	19·3	102·0	19·8	103·9	22·3
11	251	77·4	20·7	90·2	18·9	99·4	17·6	103·1	18·5	104·1	20·5
12	304	76·7	20·7	87·5	19·0	97·5	17·5	100·4	18·7	101·3	21·5
13	336	77·1	20·4	89·0	18·7	98·4	17·6	101·7	17·5	103·6	19·8
14	345	72·1	22·6	83·5	20·9	93·7	19·3	98·7	20·2	101·0	21·5
15	351	74·9	20·2	86·7	17·8	96·6	17·3	100·5	19·7	103·1	21·5
16	194	76·4	21·2	86·5	19·0	96·5	17·5	101·1	18·0	104·6	19·6
17	36	74·8	24·7	84·1	24·8	95·2	22·2	99·7	21·0	104·5	21·5
18	29	67·4	23·0	81·2	18·7	96·8	12·8	98·2	17·9	103·5	20·6
19	2	82·5		102·5		112·0		115·0		115·0	
2–19	**2704**	**77·4**	**21·1**	**88·6**	**19·5**	**97·9**	**18·2**	**101·5**	**18·9**	**103·6**	**22·5**

1 Normal
2 Very easy to follow
3 Fairly easy to follow
4 Rather difficult to follow
5 Very difficult to follow
6 Unintelligible
7 No speech

There are one or two points arising from this procedure that require expansion and clarification. For example, the class teacher herself was asked to rate the speech intelligibility of her children. Surely it would have been more relevant to find out how the man in the street perceives the speech intelligibility of each child, rather than the class teacher whose ratings are bound to reflect an overestimation of the speech intelligibility of the children. This argument is certainly correct but its main implication, that is the use of naive listeners instead of teachers to act as judges, is not accepted in this context because it is virtually impossible to implement it with such a large number of children.

Each class teacher was asked to rate the overall speech intelligibility of

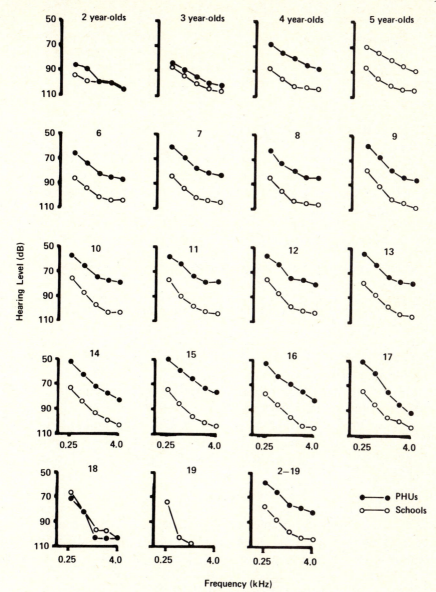

FIGURE 7.7 Average pure tone audiograms (better ear) of pupils in PHUs and in schools for the deaf

each child. This instruction could easily have been interpreted differently by individual teachers. For example, speech intelligibility under what conditions – in the classroom, on the playing field, at home, with or without a background noise, with or without contextual or environmental clues, face to face, without watching, tape-recorded speech? A very complex and very confusing situation. But that is precisely the reason why

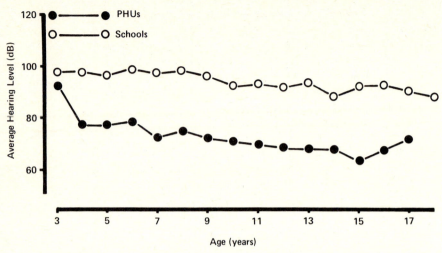

FIGURE 7.8 Average hearing levels of pupils in PHUs and in schools for the deaf

in this survey the class teachers were requested to use their intimate knowledge of each child's speech and to furnish an *overall* assessment of its intelligibility.

Of course, there are a number of limitations to this procedure. For example, no claim is made regarding the usefulness of this procedure for clinical, individual or small group comparative child study purposes. It is emphasised that the purpose of the survey was simply to establish broad national evaluative information on the speech intelligibility of hearing-impaired children as perceived by the class teachers, and to examine the relationships of rated speech intelligibility to other important character-istics of the pupils.

The methods used in this survey were deliberately planned to be quick, very simple and straightforward. This does not mean that they lack accuracy. Far from it. Simple methods of investigation are extremely powerful when used with large-scale data for the purpose of elucidating basic trends and relationships.

RATINGS OBTAINED

Tables 7.5 and 7.6 show the speech intelligibility ratings obtained expressed as a percentage of pupils falling within each speech intelligibi-lity category. The first table relates to pupils in PHUs and the second table to pupils in schools for the deaf. Similar information is shown graphically in Figures 7.9 and 7.10.

The speech intelligibility of 22·4 per cent of the pupils in PHUs was rated as 'normal', 26·1 per cent as 'very easy to follow', 19·6 per cent as 'fairly easy to follow', 13·9 per cent as 'rather difficult to follow', 10·5 per

TABLE 7.5   Speech intelligibility ratings obtained:
all pupils in PHUs

Age group in years	N	\multicolumn{7}{c}{Speech intelligibility categories % pupils}						
		1	2	3	4	5	6	7
2	4		25·0		25·0		25·0	25·0
3	52		3·8	11·5	11·5	21·2	30·8	21·2
4	79	8·9	16·5	27·8	10·1	7·6	12·7	16·5
5	132	6·8	21·2	20·5	9·8	21·2	14·4	6·1
6	166	10·8	24·7	16·9	19·3	14·5	9·6	4·2
7	153	20·3	22·9	24·8	13·7	13·7	3·3	1·3
8	200	17·0	26·0	21·0	17·0	14·0	4·0	1·0
9	199	22·6	29·1	21·1	16·1	6·5	3·5	1·0
10	216	24·1	26·9	20·8	15·3	9·3	3·7	
11	222	27·0	29·7	16·7	16·2	9·9	0·5	
12	249	22·1	27·3	22·1	14·9	8·8	3·6	1·2
13	222	26·1	28·8	20·3	9·5	10·4	4·1	0·9
14	216	30·6	28·2	17·1	13·0	7·4	3·2	0·5
15	184	35·9	31·5	13·0	9·8	4·9	3·8	1·1
16	111	32·4	23·4	18·9	11·7	9·0	4·5	
17	17	29·4	17·6	29·4	5·9	11·8	5·9	
18	6	16·7		16·7	50·0	16·7		
2–18	**2429**	**22·4**	**26·1**	**19·6**	**13·9**	**10·5**	**5·4**	**2·2**

cent as 'very difficult to follow', 5·4 per cent as 'unintelligible' and 2·2 per cent came under the last category 'no speech'. The corresponding percentage figures for the pupils in schools for the deaf were: 5·5, 15·3, 20·8, 19·5, 19·6, 12·2 and 6·9.

There was considerable variation in the distribution of these percentage figures according to age but on the whole the speech intelligibility ratings of the pupils in age groups 4 to 17 showed the same pattern. Some unusual results can be observed with the 18-year-olds where the pupils in schools for the deaf had better speech intelligibility ratings than those in PHUs, but this is mainly due to the influence of one particular school from which the great majority of the 18-year-olds were drawn.

Overall the rated speech intelligibility of the girls in both PHUs and in schools for the deaf was slightly better, but not significantly so, than that of the boys. Age did not play a major part in speech intelligibility. There was an obvious improvement up to the age of 7 but thereafter the differences were slight and none proved to be of any significant value. The correlation between age and speech intelligibility ratings was 0·01, a non-significant value. At face value, this is a disappointing result but in reality it was expected, because children of different ages were rated on differing sets of speech requirements.

TABLE 7.6 Speech intelligibility ratings obtained:
all pupils in schools for the deaf

Age group in years	N	Speech intelligibility categories % pupils						
		1	2	3	4	5	6	7
2	7						57·1	42·9
3	35		5·7	8·6	2·9	11·4	45·7	25·7
4	31		3·2		6·5	16·1	29·0	45·2
5	68	2·9	7·4	30·9	4·4	20·6	17·6	16·2
6	104	1·9	8·7	18·3	19·2	20·2	21·2	10·6
7	137	3·6	6·6	20·4	19·7	23·4	13·1	13·1
8	135	3·7	7·4	15·6	23·7	25·9	12·6	11·1
9	162	6·2	13·0	14·2	22·2	25·9	12·3	5·6
10	216	6·5	13·0	22·7	20·8	15·3	12·0	9·7
11	251	6·4	17·5	22·3	21·5	16·7	11·2	4·4
12	304	5·3	19·1	22·7	23·7	18·4	7·2	3·6
13	336	5·4	11·9	23·5	21·1	18·8	12·5	6·8
14	345	4·1	22·6	22·9	17·4	20·0	9·3	3·8
15	351	6·3	17·7	20·5	18·2	20·5	13·4	3·4
16	194	7·2	20·1	19·6	19·1	21·6	9·3	3·1
17	36	16·7	11·1	27·8	19·4	13·9	5·6	5·6
18	29	27·6	34·5	13·8	13·8	6·9	6·9	
2–18	**2743**	**5·5**	**15·3**	**30·8**	**19·5**	**19·6**	**12·2**	**6·9**

DEGREE OF HEARING LOSS AND RATED SPEECH INTELLIGIBILITY

Table 7.7 and Figure 7.11 show the distribution of the speech intelligibility ratings obtained according to the average hearing levels (AHL) of the
pupils. AHL were calculated by averaging the hearing levels in the better
ear of each pupil across the frequencies 250 Hz to 4000 Hz. The 'no
responses' in any one of these frequencies were entered as 120 dB and for
those children without a pure tone audiogram (1·1%) the AHL was based
on their reported responses to meaningful sound stimuli such as speech
and high frequency rattle.

Note that the speech intelligibility of the pupils in each hearing loss
group was distributed throughout the seven speech intelligibility categories. These distributions, however, varied considerably with degree of
hearing loss. The maximum concentration of pupils in the speech
intelligibility distributions in each hearing loss group is shown in bold
type in Table 7.7. These maximum figures correspond to the peaks of the
speech intelligibility distributions as shown in Figure 7.11.

As expected the speech intelligibility of the pupils deteriorated with
increasing degree of hearing loss. The picture emerging is as follows: AHL
50 dB or below, highest concentration of pupils under speech intelligibi-

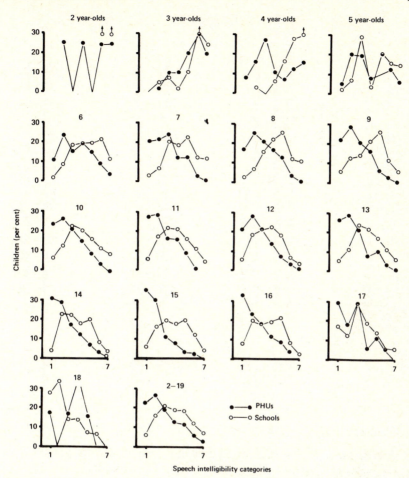

FIGURE 7.9 Distribution of speech intelligibility ratings by age: pupils in PHUs and in schools for the deaf

lity category 1 (normal); AHL 51 dB to 80 dB, highest concentration of pupils under speech intelligibility category 2 (very easy to follow); AHL 81 dB to 100 dB, highest concentration of pupils under speech intelligibility category 3 (fairly easy to follow); and AHL 101 dB to 120 dB, highest concentration of pupils under speech category 5 (very difficult to follow). Of course these figures do not tell the whole story but the details can easily be seen in Table 7.7 and Figure 7.11. The correlation between AHL and speech intelligibility ratings was −0·62.

ADDITIONAL HANDICAP AND RATED SPEECH INTELLIGIBILITY

As stated previously a considerable number of hearing-impaired pupils both in the PHUs and in the schools for the deaf suffered from one or

SPEECH INTELLIGIBILITY CATEGORIES

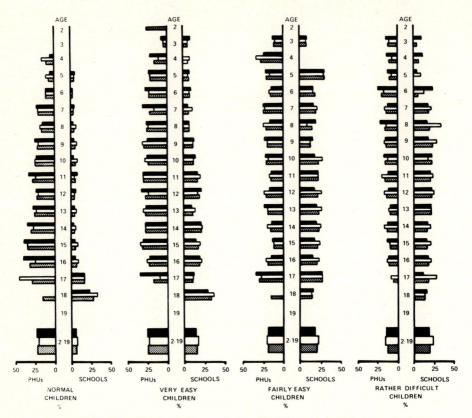

FIGURE 7.10 Distribution of speech intelligibility ratings by age and sex:
pupils in PHUs and in schools for the deaf

more handicaps in addition to deafness. It was decided, therefore, to look into the rated speech intelligibility of these pupils and to compare it with the speech intelligibility ratings of the hearing-impaired pupils who were not reported to have any additional handicaps. These comparisons were carried out within four major hearing loss categories and the results are presented in Figure 7.12.

The speech intelligibility of the hearing-impaired pupils with additional handicap was significantly inferior ($p = 0.01$) to that of the hearing-impaired pupils who were not suffering from additional handicap. This was true in all four hearing loss categories.

FOLLOW UP

During the period of carrying out this survey a number of teachers of the deaf both from PHUs and schools for the deaf have written to the author

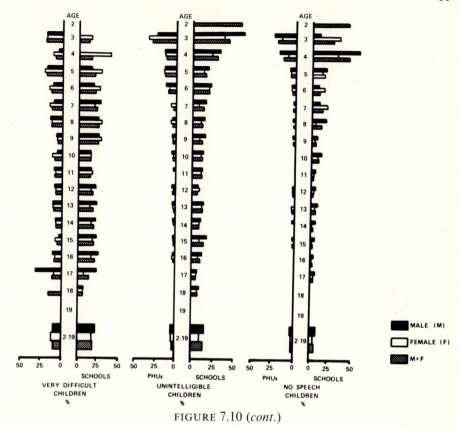

FIGURE 7.10 (*cont.*)

raising a number of very pertinent questions. Two questions in particular kept cropping up. The first one related to the validity and repeatability of the speech ratings obtained, and the second question queried the advisability of using class teachers instead of inexperienced listeners to act as judges or assessors.

With regard to the first question, the author visited one school for the deaf and three PHUs, the teachers of which were concerned about this and requested them to repeat their ratings. In particular the teachers concerned were carefully instructed to use the same scale and to rate the *overall* speech intelligibility of their pupils, *as perceived by them*, taking into consideration factors such as: with or without contextual clues, face to face, listening only, speech intelligibility within the classroom, in the playground, etc. Their second assessment ratings, together with their original ones, are shown in Figure 7.13 C and D. The repeatability of ratings among these teachers was extremely high ($r=0.97$) and this strengthens considerably the validity of the initial ratings obtained.

With regard to the second question the same teachers were also requested to undertake a third assessment of speech intelligibility of their

TABLE 7.7   Degree of hearing loss and rated speech intelligibility

Average hearing level in dB	Speech intelligibility categories Number of children							Row total	Cumulative %
	1	2	3	4	5	6	7		
≤30	55	27	12	6	3	1	3	107 2.1%	2.1
31–40	96	39	9	7	3	1	0	155 3.0%	5.1
41–50	148	97	46	10	5	3	4	313 6.1%	11.2
51–60	144	155	81	15	7	2	3	407 7.9%	19.1
61–70	93	206	105	45	14	3	7	473 9.1%	28.2
71–80	71	181	167	81	41	10	7	558 10.8%	39.0
81–90	51	167	204	121	79	34	21	677 13.0%	52.0
91–100	26	119	231	229	204	112	40	961 18.6%	70.6
101–110	6	56	153	275	307	184	73	1054 20.4%	91.0
111–120	5	9	38	84	131	116	84	467 9.0%	100.0
Column total	695 13.4%	1056 20.4%	1046 20.2%	873 16.9%	794 15.4%	466 9.0%	242 4.7%	5172 100.0%	
Cumulative %	13.4	33.8	54.0	70.9	86.3	95.3	100.0		

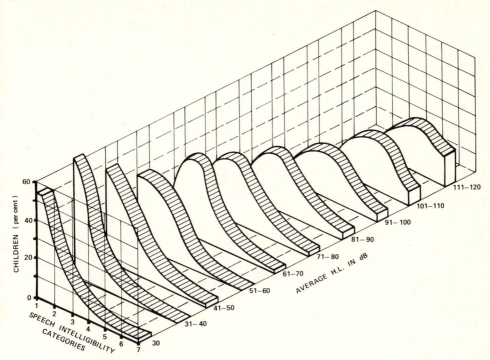

FIGURE 7.11 Distribution of speech intelligibility ratings by degree of hearing loss: pupils in PHUs and in schools for the deaf

pupils, but on this occasion they were asked to put themselves in the place of an inexperienced listener. In detail they were instructed as follows:

Please put yourself in the place of a helpful normally hearing shopkeeper. Each one of your pupils goes into the shop and asks orally to buy a number of things, such as a bag of crisps, chocolate, a pound of apples, a loaf of bread, Coca-Cola etc. How well do you think the shopkeeper would understand the speech of the child?

The ratings obtained for the third assessment are shown in Figure 7.13 C and D. Note that the differences in ratings obtained were primarily concentrated in speech intelligibility categories 2 and 3. The same pattern was also evident in the 1967 study where both teachers and inexperienced assessors were asked to rate the tape-recorded speech of hearing-impaired children (Figure 7.13 A and B).

These two sets of results have shown a similar relationship between the ratings of experienced and 'inexperienced' listeners, with the latter finding the speech of hearing-impaired children more difficult to understand. This, of course, was expected but the most important thing here is the relationship between the two sets of ratings. Once this relationship is

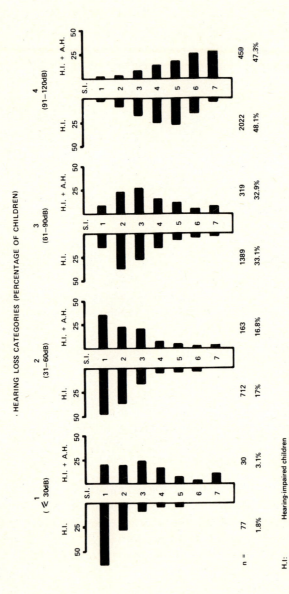

FIGURE 7.12 Distribution of speech intelligibility ratings: hearing-impaired pupils v hearing-impaired pupils with additional handicaps

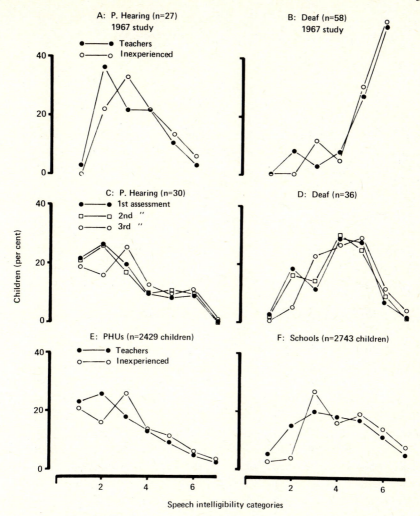

FIGURE 7.13 Distribution of speech intelligibility ratings: experienced v inexperienced listeners

known then it is very easy to extrapolate from one set of ratings to another. This has been done and the resulting information as to how the speech intelligibility ratings of the pupils in this survey would have been distributed had the assessors been inexperienced listeners is shown in Figure 7.13 E and F.

One can, of course, argue that this is a poor substitute for the real thing, that is having inexperienced assessors for each one of the pupils taking part. As stated previously, this is certainly a very valid point when dealing with a small number of children but it is virtually impossible to implement when dealing with thousands of pupils. Furthermore, the purpose of the survey was to find out what the *class teachers themselves* thought of the speech intelligibility of their pupils, not anybody else.

DISCUSSION

The purpose of this national survey was to find out what the class teachers themselves thought of the speech intelligibility of their pupils. Overall, the survey collected relevant information on 5172 hearing-impaired pupils, 2429 of them attending 272 PHUs and 2743 from 44 schools for the deaf. These figures could not have been achieved without the goodwill, support and professionalism of the British teachers of the deaf. Their response, especially when seen in conjunction with the constraints of time imposed on them, can only be described as magnificent. From these figures it can be stated that the pupils involved in the survey are representative of the entire British hearing-impaired pupil population attending schools for the deaf and PHUs.

Several important pupil characteristics emerged. The first related to the rapid decline in numbers of hearing-impaired children attending schools for the deaf and it was postulated that if the same trend continued for another five to ten years, then quite a large proportion of the existing schools for the deaf would find it very difficult to continue functioning. Furthermore, there is a growing tendency to send a proportionally increasing number of hearing-impaired children into local PHUs for their primary education and this, of course, deprives schools for the deaf of potential pupils. There is no doubt that educating hearing-impaired children in PHUs is certainly a very desirable development, provided the education offered in these units meets the needs and potentials of the pupils attending them. This is not always the case. It is the author's opinion that the number of hearing-impaired children who are educationally 'misplaced' in units is at present substantial and it is constantly growing.

The second characteristic related to the causes of deafness reported. In 50 per cent of all pupils involved in the survey, cause of deafness was unknown. This is a very high figure that needs to be reduced drastically. Contrary to popular belief, rubella is still the major known cause of deafness in children and there is no sign that this is substantially changing.

The third important pupil characteristic emerging related to the prevalence of additional handicaps. As stated, 16·3 per cent of the pupils in PHUs and 20·9 per cent of the pupils in schools for the deaf had one or more handicaps in addition to hearing loss. This is quite a high proportion of pupils especially when one considers that in some schools for the deaf the figure is as high as 90 per cent.

The fourth characteristic related to the degree of hearing loss of the pupils. On average the degree of hearing loss of the children admitted into schools for the deaf at present is more severe than that of the children admitted five or ten years ago. The same applies to children in PHUs.

Overall then the hearing-impaired pupil population of both PHUs and schools for the deaf is changing, not only in declining numbers but also in important characteristics such as additional handicap and severity of hearing loss. These changes are bound to affect educational standards in schools for the deaf.

With regard to the rated speech intelligibility of the pupils the following facts emerged. If one considers the first three speech intelligibility categories as 'functional' or 'socially acceptable' then on average nearly 70 per cent of all pupils (range 50–80% by age) and just over 40 per cent (range 25–55% by age) of all pupils in schools for the deaf fall within this grouping. Bearing in mind the limitations of these children, brought about primarily as a result of deafness and also additional handicaps, these figures are a testimony to the endeavours and perseverance of the children, their parents and their teachers. Of course, there is still room for considerable improvement, and such an improvement can, to a large extent, be achieved through more intensive, systematic and consistent speech teaching.

The most important variable affecting the speech intelligibility of the hearing-impaired pupils was the degree of hearing loss. As hearing loss increased speech intelligibility became worse ($r = -0.62$). The distribution of the speech intelligibility ratings within each hearing loss group highlighted the fact that some children in spite of very severe hearing loss still managed to acquire perfectly normal speech intelligibility. It would be most interesting to study these children in detail with a view to identifying contributing factors.

This survey provides valuable information on hearing-impaired pupils attending PHUs and schools for the deaf throughout the UK. A similar survey in twenty, thirty or more years will undoubtedly prove to be a most fascinating comparative study.

PART III

Speech for the hearing-impaired child:
scientific base; principles, objectives and strategies

'Looky here, Jim; . . . ain't it natural and right for a cat and a cow to talk different from *us*?'

'Why, mos' sholy it is.'

'Well, then, why ain't it natural and right for a *Frenchman* to talk different from us? You answer me that.'

'Is a cat a man, Huck?'

'No.'

'Well, den, dey ain't no sense in a cat talkin' like a man. Is a cow a man? – er is a cow a cat?'

'No, she ain't either of them.'

'Well, den, she ain't got no business to talk like either one er the yuther of 'em. Is a Frenchman a man?'

'Yes.'

'*Well*, den! Dad blame it, why doan' he *talk* like a man? You answer me *dat*!'

Mark Twain: *The Adventures of Huckleberry Finn*

CHAPTER EIGHT

Speech development and speech perceptual processes: hearing children

The average hearing child, despite ill health, social privations, unfavourable home background and limited exposure to speech, is still able to mobilise his natural resources and achieve acceptable speech skills.

Speech acquisition begins shortly after birth and thereafter grows at a fast rate both in quantity and in complexity, passing through various overlapping stages (Table 8.1). The feat involved is enormous and recently Fry (1977), writing on this concluded that the more one discovers about normal speech development, the more one is inclined to favour the 'miracle theory'.

The process begins with the production of reflex vocal sounds which all babies give, whether hearing or deaf. These sounds may not be emotionally or socially meaningful but the child is using basic neuromotor coordinations, respiration and phonation, which will later provide the basis for speech production. His vocalisations contain both changes in pitch and intensity and help the child to hear his own voice, thus marking the beginning of a monitoring circuit. Soon these vocalisations develop into intentional babbling whereby the child produces a considerable variety of sounds which in turn reinforce further the complex motor and auditory activities. As he begins to perceive the phonological components of speech, imitation becomes of primary importance. The child begins to copy the sounds made to him by adults, especially his mother, and then imposes them on his intonational patterns, first in babbling and then in jargon, in words and phrases and finally in sentences. During this process he masters the prosody of his mother tongue, he arranges his speech into appropriate breath intervals, he develops full articulatory competence, he learns the rules according to which morphemes and words are put together to form sentences, he acquires an extensive vocabulary and associates speech with meaning. In other words, within a very short period of time the normal child gains command of the complex phonemic,

TABLE 8.1 Composite table of important stages in normal speech development in children during the first two years of life reported in major studies. (Gessel, 1940; Lewis, 1951; Miller, 1951; Griffiths, 1954; Illingworth, 1960; Watts, 1960; McCarthy, 1970)

Months

Stage of speech development	0	6	12	18	24	30
Reflex vocalisations						
Responds to human voice						
Intentional babbling						
Imitates sounds						
First word						
Conversational jargon						
Comprehends simple commands						
Imitates syllables and words						
Names object or picture						
Combines words						
Uses phrases and sentences						

syntactic and semantic system of his native language with all the intonational and articulatory expertise which that entails.

Nearly every normal child develops these abilities, without any conscious effort or imposed practice by the time he is 3 or 4 years old, primarily as a result of continual auditory stimulation, incessant exposure to speech, unceasing encouragement and hours and hours of practice. He learns, controls and perfects speech production by means of interrelated cyclical processes or feedback circuits, the most important being the auditory, kinaesthetic and tactual feedback. These three feedback loops facilitate control, timing and coordination of the complex muscle systems involved in the production of intelligible speech.

The auditory feedback circuit is by far the most essential in the learning of speech skills. Its function, although very complicated, can easily be understood by the following example. In speech the sound waves produced are also fed back into the ears of the speaker. The hearing sensations aroused are used by the brain to control the actions of all the muscles involved in speech. For example, the tongue is set moving in a particular direction and as it moves it continually brings about changes in the sound reaching the speaker's ears. These changes are constantly monitored by the brain of the speaker and when the sound acquires a particular quality the necessary instructions, either to change direction or to stop, are transmitted to the tongue. In the same way the speaker controls the muscles involved in the production of pitch and loudness.

The function of the auditory feedback loop is supplemented by kinaesthetic feedback, especially in the control of speech movements. The brain receives constant information on the activities of the speech muscles and this information is used in turn to control or modify their actions. Kinaesthetic feedback depends entirely on proprioception and it must not be confused with tactual feedback which also plays an important role in the control of speech movements. Tactual feedback refers primarily to those sensations received by the speaker which are particularly connected with the movements of the tongue and the lips.

SPEECH PERCEPTUAL PROCESSES

According to Hirsh (1965) speech perception is the process that takes place when listeners seem to understand what is said to them. Such a process is a complicated one, being dependent upon physiological, acoustical and linguistic factors which are intrinsically interwoven. The physiological factors involved have been well documented by Denes and Pinson (1963) and by Whetnall and Fry (1964). The physical factors have been widely researched and their unique contribution to speech perception will be dealt with later on. First of all, however, it is intended to present the linguistic factors, mainly because they are seldom given the attention they deserve.

For effective communication to occur between two people through the medium of speech, a common knowledge of the same language is essential. Our knowledge of the language helps us to fill in any gaps that may occur in the stream of words we hear. In 1949, Shannon, using his 'guessing' technique, demonstrated very clearly that we possess an extensive knowledge of the statistics of our language, so much so that even if we only hear half of what is spoken we have no difficulty at all in guessing the rest of it, making practically no mistakes. The high degree of predictability of phonemes or of words in a sentence fluctuates as the sequence proceeds, since it is dependent on the number of possible choices at any given position (Fry, 1963). The operation of sequential probabilities has been highlighted by Denes and Pinson (1963) and Fry (1964). They carried out similar experiments and reached similar conclusions. For example, Fry selected at random a sentence and asked a person to guess its first phoneme. He counted the number of mistakes made before the person found the right phoneme and then repeated the same procedure for the second phoneme and so on. He found that nearly half of the phonemes were guessed correctly at the first go. This shows that we recognise many phonemes without the help of acoustic cues. We recognise them because we know the language; we know its phonemes and the way they may or may not combine; we know its words and the way they may or may not be strung together. In other words, we know its vocabulary, its grammar and its semantics. We quickly gather the meaning of what is being said and, more often than not, we are able to anticipate what is going to follow and our success in anticipating increases dramatically as the linguistic sequence progresses (Denes, 1963).

The acoustical factors operating in the perception of speech sounds can be thought of broadly as belonging to the frequency domain, the intensity domain and the time domain (Cherry, 1961). Of course, such a classification is an oversimplification, since acoustically the three domains interpenetrate. Nevertheless this categorisation provides a practical framework within which the different acoustic cues used in speech perception can be discussed.

Frequency domain
The acoustic cues operating in the recognition of English vowels, for

example, fall mainly in the frequency domain. Vowel recognition depends mainly on the ability of the listener to distinguish, first the position in frequency of the first two formants, secondly the relation between them and thirdly the relations of $F1/F2$ frequencies for all the vowels in the system (Broadbent and Ladefoged, 1960).

Frequency cues also operate in the recognition of consonants. Nasal consonants for example, are characterised by a peak of energy which occurs at a low frequency, around 500 Hz, with a very weak $F2$ followed by a relatively strong $F3$. Studies with synthetic speech (Delattre, Libernam and Cooper, 1955; Hughes and Halle, 1956; Stevens, 1960) established two types of acoustic cues for the perception of consonantal place of production. One relates to the position on the frequency scale of the peaks of energy or friction produced. When dealing with plosive consonants, for example, a low frequency peak (300–400 Hz) indicates /p, b/, a mid-frequency peak (1500–2000 Hz) /k, g/, and a high frequency peak around 4000 Hz /t, d/. Harris (1958) showed that the same principle also operates with the fricatives. The /s/ sound, for example, covers a frequency spectrum from about 4000 to 6500 Hz, while the acoustic energy for /ʃ/ starts much lower, from about 1500 Hz and falls away around 6000 Hz.

Intensity domain

Not only do intensity differences contribute to differentiating vowels from consonants (the former being more intense than the latter), but also such differences provide important cues in differentiating among vowels and also among consonants. For example, intensity provides the most important cue for discriminating between voiced and voiceless consonants (Fry, 1964). In voiced sounds the burst of acoustic energy is of higher intensity than in voiceless sounds. Also, intensity differences contribute to the differentiation of the fricatives according to their place of production; /s/ and /ʃ/ are high intensity sounds, /f/ and /θ/ are low intensity sounds.

Time domain

The relative duration of the different English vowels provides the main cue for distinction between long and short vowels, especially when dealing with vowels with similar intensity and frequency parameters. The recognition of a sound as belonging either to the plosive or fricative group is brought about mainly by time cues. In plosives, for example, these time cues relate first to the short silence that takes place during the temporary closure of the oral passage and secondly to the short burst of acoustic energy that follows the sudden release of the closure. Contrary to this, the fricative group is characterised by random acoustic energy of considerable duration.

Also relatively rapid changes in frequency or formant transitions provide important cues in speech perception. These transitions can be adequately described by reference either to the point on the frequency scale at which the transition originates or to that which it may be said to point to. The term 'minus transition' is used when the transition is to or from a frequency below that of the main formant and 'plus transition' when the transition is to or from a frequency above that of the main formant (Delattre, Liberman and Cooper, 1955).

Transitions of the second and sometimes third formant are important cues for place of articulation. This depends primarily on the direction and extent of the frequency shift. A minus $F2$ transition, for example, indicates labials /p, b, m/, a marked plus $F2$ transition is associated with velars /k, g, ŋ/, and a slight plus or no $F2$ transition indicates alveolar place of articulation /t, d, n/ (Stevens and House, 1955; O'Connor, Liberman, Delattre and Cooper, 1957; Harris, 1958; Hoffman, 1958).

Harris (1958) showed that the differentiation between /f/ and /θ/ sounds depends primarily on the $F2$ transition of the periodic sound preceding or following these consonants. Periodic sounds associated with /f/ have a marked minus transition of $F2$ while there is no $F2$ transition or only a slight one with /θ/. The $F2$ and $F3$ transitions of the laterals and semi-vowels /l, r, w, j/ are extremely slow when compared to those associated with plosives. The former last from about 60 to 100 ms, whilst the latter take around 40 ms.

Influence of adjacent sounds

Speech sounds seldom occur in isolation; they are nearly always strung together to form words. In any combination of sounds there is a tendency for each one of them to be influenced by its neighbours (Liberman, Delattre and Cooper, 1952; Delattre, Liberman and Cooper, 1955). Suffice it to say that sounds carry more than one kind of acoustical information about themselves and their neighbours and that the exact interpretation of this acoustical information depends on context (Broadbent and Ladefoged, 1960).

SUMMARY

It is evident that the production of speech is very closely interwoven with the reception of speech, so much so that the two processes in the young child go forward together and are inseparably connected. From the very beginning both the amount of speech the child hears and also the environment and circumstances under which the child hears speech form the basis for his future verbal development.

The importance of audition in the perception and development of speech is paramount. It is not surprising therefore that throughout the ages and especially in the last century great efforts have been made to maximise the use of the residual hearing of hearing-impaired children. As we shall see in the next chapter, however, speech perception in the hearing-impaired child is greatly enhanced when auditory cues are supported by cues from other modalities such as vision and vibrotaction.

CHAPTER NINE

Speech development and speech perceptual processes: hearing-impaired children

Right from the very beginning the hearing-impaired child suffers limitations in all areas vital to speech development. A hearing impairment interferes partially or totally, depending on its severity, with auditory feedback. Interference with this autocorrective cyclical process affects both the quantity and clarity of the speech reaching the hearing-impaired child. In addition, the child may fail to hear himself. He ceases to babble and fails to enter the jargon stage. He is unable to monitor his own vocal output and therefore fails to develop and experience the right tactile and kinaesthetic sensations which eventually will enable him to master the complex movements of speech, including breath control. This leads to inappropriate use of the speech organs – their control is affected and this can bring about changes in their physical structure and development (Holm, 1970). The child's environment is also severely modified. The pleasures of speech, the 'emotionality' of speech, the psychological and social aspects of speech may fail to reach the hearing-impaired child. His handicap may cause great strain and stress for his parents and this in turn may influence both their attitudes and their linguistic behaviour towards him. Speech and language do not develop in the normal fashion. The child affected has to learn his speech and language through faulty auditory channels which receive, comparatively speaking, very little stimulation and which, most probably, are highly distorted. In addition to these difficulties which arise either directly or indirectly from a hearing impairment, one must not overlook the possibility that whatever caused the hearing damage could also have caused further damage impinging on central processes in speech perception, i.e. integration problems, difficulties in selective attention and short-term memory. These disabilities are not easily detectable, especially when they are clouded by an obvious hearing impairment. We have a fairly good idea of the handicapping effects of deafness on speech development. The question arising of course is: what can we do about it? The following is an attempt to answer this question.

USE OF AUDITION

It is generally accepted that all hearing-impaired children can respond to sound if it is sufficiently intense. In most cases these responses are an indication of residual auditory sensitivity, while in some they may be due solely to vibrotactile stimulation (Boothroyd and Cawkwell, 1970). With suitable amplification equipment the great majority of hearing-impaired children can be helped to establish a functional auditory feedback process which, in the most favourable instances, will enable them to recognise and monitor speech sounds and in the least favourable, will at least convey some of the prosodic aspects of speech.

EARLY AUDITORY STIMULATION

The importance of audition in learning to speak is paramount and it has already been highlighted. Perhaps what needs to be emphasised here is the need to establish this auditory feedback process as soon as possible following the onset of deafness and, for those children born deaf, preferably within their first six months of life. The latter part of this recommendation may be very difficult to achieve mainly because at present, even in the most advanced countries in the world, it is very difficult to ascertain and diagnose deafness in children during their first six months. With the rapid development of computerised techniques in auditory investigations, however, it will not be long before early diagnosis of deafness becomes a reality. The early restoration of auditory feedback is recommended mainly because the cumulative writings of linguistic researchers in the last five decades point to this period, the first six months of life, as a crucial period for speech development. They point to the fact that it is mainly within this period that most children change their reflex vocalisations to intentional babbling which forms the basis for subsequent speech development. Failure to accomplish this change results in severe speech retardation. The degree of success in restoring the auditory feedback process will of course depend both on the residual capacity of the child to hear and on the amplification equipment used.

RESIDUAL CAPACITY TO HEAR

An indication of the child's residual capacity to hear speech can be obtained, to a certain extent, by examining his pure tone audiogram. It needs to be stressed, however, that such an examination has limited value because the pure tone audiogram does not provide reliable information as to how well the child's hearing functions above threshold. The only way of finding this out is to administer speech discrimination tests at several suprathreshold levels. The great majority of hearing-impaired children will be able to cooperate in speech discrimination testing. Some of them, however, either because of age or other developmental factors, will not be able to do so and therefore reliance on the pure tone audiogram may be essential.

The information previously presented on the normal processes in auditory speech perception gives an indication of the potential for children with a hearing impairment. For example, even a child without any residual hearing but with some vibrotactile sensitivity should be able to distinguish temporal patterns in speech and to differentiate between voiced and unvoiced sounds (Nober, 1967; Risberg, 1968; Erber, 1972). A child with residual hearing up to 250 Hz can receive valuable auditory information especially on the suprasegmental aspects of speech. A child with sensitivity up to 1000 Hz can potentially detect most suprasegmental features of speech; one or more formants of all vowels; the voiced–voiceless distinction and, in combination with lipreading, all manner of distinctions between consonants. When hearing extends to 3000 Hz the second formant is audible. This provides accurate differentiation between most vowels and also enhances the recognition of most consonants. A child with hearing up to 4000 Hz is usually able to process most speech patterns through hearing alone, provided of course, he is using the correct amplification and is trained to do so.

USE OF RESIDUAL HEARING

Unfortunately, even at present, it is not unusual to come across hearing-impaired children who are using individual hearing aids that do not meet their needs, especially in terms of acoustic output and frequency response. Before considering these two basic electroacoustic properties of hearing aids it is pertinent to mention here two particular modes of hearing aid amplification that have been found to have considerable advantages. These modes of amplification are binaural hearing aids and radio hearing aids.

Binaural hearing aids, be they ear-level or bodyworn, facilitate speech discrimination and also dramatically enhance localisation ability. The first benefit directly affects social intercourse by improving communication ability. Improvement in localisation helps the child to establish the association between sounds and objects, actions and circumstances, and to externalise the source of the sound and locate it in space with accuracy. The benefits to the child stemming from this enhanced ability in terms of linguistic development, psychological and physical well-being and general awareness of his environment can be enormous. Most hearing-impaired children are suitable candidates for binaural hearing aids. It is not intended to go into details on selection procedures here – this has been dealt with elsewhere (Markides, 1977).

Radio hearing aids when selectively used, especially when used in combination with the individual hearing aids of the children, are extremely effective for speech reception. With radio hearing aids the microphone is near the mouth of the speaker, thus providing a better speech input in terms of signal-to-noise ratio. It is advisable, however, not to use radio hearing aids constantly because by doing so the children are denied important localisation clues.

Acoustic output

A hearing aid is expected to provide a sufficiently high level of acoustic output to enable hearing-impaired children to hear speech at adequate levels above their thresholds. The MRC report (1947) concluded that the needs of most deaf people could be met with a hearing aid having undistorted maximum output of 120 dB (rms re 20 μPa). The Harvard report (Hudgins et al., 1948) proposed 132 dB with variant maximum settings at 126, 120 and 114 dB. Rice (1965) was of the opinion that the maximum output level of a hearing aid should be restricted to 125 dB provided enough amplification was given in the 250–750 Hz frequency range. Watson (1967) preferred 130–135 dB as the maximum output level of a hearing aid.

McCandless (1976) looked upon this problem in terms of gain requirements and suggested individual gain settings equivalent to approximately 50 per cent of the hearing deficit. Gengel (1974) determined that the user gain averaged 20–25 dB above detection threshold. Similar recommendations, based on a wide variety of formulae, were put forward by several other workers such as Brooks (1973), Martin (1973) and Morris (1975). These formulae may have some merits but they have severe limitations too (Markides, 1980c). Suffice it to state here that none of the published formulae on this matter meets the individual requirements of each child.

It is difficult to be specific regarding clearcut maximum output levels or gain specifications of hearing aids. Indeed such a question can only be answered on an individual basis. It is accepted, however, that the needs of the great majority of children suffering from sensorineural hearing losses can be met with wearable hearing aids having maximum acoustic outputs ranging from 110 to 130 dB SPL. For children with severe hearing losses, 110–120 dB, outputs well in excess of 130 dB SPL may be required. By contrast, some children need special 'lower-power' aids since many aids provide too much amplification for them even at the lowest end of the aid's gain setting.

The question arises, of course, as to whether powerful hearing aids cause further deterioration of hearing. Works by Kinney (1953, 1961), Møller and Rojskjaer (1960), Sataloff (1961), Ross and Truex (1965), Macrae and Farrant (1965), Ross and Lerman (1967), Macrae (1967, 1968) and Ballantyne (1970) uphold the idea that powerful hearing aids have a deleterious effect on the user's residual hearing. The opposite view was put forward by Holmgren (1940), Murray (1951), Naunton (1957), Brockman (1959), Whetnall (1964), Barr and Wedenberg (1965), World Health Organisation (1967), Bellefluer and Van Dyke (1968), Roberts (1970), Hine and Furness (1975) and Darbyshire (1976). Markides (1971, 1976) and Markides and Aryee (1978, 1980) in a longitudinal study stretching over a period of 6 years did not find any deterioration of hearing that could have been reasonably attributed to the use of powerful hearing aids. They did advocate caution, however.

Frequency response

With regard to frequency response it is of interest to recall that the MRC report recommended that the most useful frequency range of an aid was from 250 to 4000 Hz. Similarly the Harvard report recommended a frequency range from 300 to 4000 Hz. Hudgins and his associates (1948), however, recommended a hearing aid with wider frequency response characteristics than those put forward in the above-mentioned reports. Watson (1956) and Olsen and Carhart (1967) preferred hearing aids with relatively flat frequency response characteristics extending up to at least 6000 Hz.

The frequency response characteristics proposed by the MRC and Harvard reports provided limited amplification in the low frequencies. Wedenberg (1954) and later Huizing (1959) pointed out that most hearing-impaired children have better residual hearing in the frequency region below 750 Hz. It is also recalled that vocal cord vibrations are low fundamental frequencies and carry important information especially on the suprasegmental aspects of speech. It was with these views in mind that Ling (1964), Rice (1965) and Brinskey and Sinclair (1966) recommended the use of hearing aids with extended low frequency amplification down to about 100 Hz. It is true that excessive low frequency amplification in some instances may have some adverse effects on the perception of high frequency sounds mainly because of an upward spread of masking. The advantages to be gained from extended low frequency amplification, however, greatly outweigh the disadvantages. It is pertinent to note here that during the tabulation of the results of the national survey on speech intelligibility, reported in Chapter 7, it was observed that those children with good residual hearing at 250 Hz (30–60 dB) were consistently rated as having speech intelligibility that was normal, very easy or fairly easy to follow. This relationship between residual hearing at 250 Hz and speech intelligibility is currently being looked at in more detail and the results will be reported in due course. The evidence so far collected, however, consistently points to the great importance of low frequency amplification with regard to speech intelligibility.

In summary, it can be stated that individual hearing aids should provide sufficient undistorted amplification to enable hearing-impaired children to hear speech at adequate levels above their detection threshold and they should also provide a wide frequency response, preferably from 100 Hz to at least 4000 Hz.

It is emphasised that the efficiency of all hearing aids is greatly affected by the influence of environmental factors such as noise background, reverberation and the distance and direction of the speaker from the microphone.

Noise background

The influence of background noise on speech perception through hearing aids has been well documented by Tillman, Carhart and Olsen (1970). They found that while normal hearing subjects could achieve 40 per cent discrimination even when the signal was 12 dB less intense than the noise, hearing-impaired subjects required the signal to be 18 dB greater than the competing noise to achieve the same level of discrimination, a 30 dB difference. Extraneous noises can be avoided with careful acoustic insulation. Unwanted sounds generated within a room can be dealt with through noise-reducing floor coverings and materials fixed to the base of movable objects.

Reverberation

Under normal environmental conditions the detrimental effects of background noise are compounded by room reverberation. John (1957) reported that with a reverberation time of 0·7 seconds discrimination scores of only 52 per cent were achieved by a group of deafened adults, whereas with a reduction in reverberation time to 0·5 seconds their scores increased to 70 per cent. Similar results, confirming the fact that speech discrimination decreases as reverberation time increases and that hearing-impaired people are more vulnerable to the combined effects of reverberation and background noise, have been reported by Sanders (1961), Nabelek and Pickett (1974) and more recently by Nabelek (1980). The cumulative writings of these authors and others point to the fact that the optimum classroom reverberation time should not exceed 0·5 seconds.

The obvious way to reduce reverberation time is by careful sound treatment of a room. This needs to be achieved through skilful placement and choice of the sound-absorbent materials. If such materials are concentrated in certain areas of the room, the desired effect may not be achieved. Moreover, some materials absorb high frequency sounds too effectively, thus removing from speech the very acoustic clues that are essential for intelligibility.

Microphone position

A simple way of reducing the detrimental effects of both reverberation and background noise is by speaking close to the microphone of the hearing aid and preferably at a distance of not more than 10 to 15 cm. Only a quiet conversational voice is needed at this distance and the hearing aid user receives the benefit of the direct sound, thus improving the speech-to-noise ratio and at the same time reducing the effects of reverberation. In 1964 Watson, in a study designed to take into consideration the overall effect of the frequency limitations of hearing aids, the poor acoustic conditions, the noise background and the distance of the speaker from the microphone, observed a dramatic reduction in discrimination scores from 84·8 per cent in good acoustic conditions down to 35·2 per cent in conditions with ambient noise between 55 and 60 dB.

The implications of these findings for the development of good intelligible speech are clear. Each hearing-impaired child must listen under optimal acoustic conditions. The amplification equipment required for speech teaching purposes must be carefully selected and competently used. The children's individual hearing aids, most of them with non-directional microphones, are not acceptable for this purpose. Not only do they provide restricted frequency amplification but also their microphones are situated further away than the recommended distance of 10 to 15 cm. Radio hearing aids will certainly improve this situation but in most models their frequency response characteristics are not sufficiently wide for optimal speech discrimination enhancement. Their advantages in terms of child mobility and flexibility of use, however, make them extremely effective, especially for classroom teaching. For individual speech teaching the most effective amplification equipment is undoubtedly the speech training unit (STU). For group speech teaching, especially with older children, the effectiveness of the wired group hearing aid (GHA) must not be underestimated. The electroacoustic properties of these last two pieces of equipment are very similar. They provide sufficient amplification to meet the acoustic potential of almost all hearing-impaired children. They amplify a wide range of frequencies, from as low as 100 Hz to as high as 8000 Hz. The speaker-microphone positions for both teacher and child can be arranged to be within the recommended distances, thus enhancing the speech-to-noise ratio and at the same time reducing the effects of competing background noise (Markides, Huntington and Kettlety, 1980; Fitzgerald and Markides, 1982).

There is evidence to suggest, however, that these types of amplification equipment (STUs, GHAs) are substantially misused, thus limiting their potential value (Markides, in preparation *b*). One of the major factors that contributes to misuse relates to the fact that different models and types of such equipment may not be calibrated on the same basis. For example, the same dial reading in dB can vary from one type of STU to another by as much as 20 dB SPL (Martin, 1979). The same applies to GHAs. This discrepancy leads to serious mistakes in use, especially regarding the selection of the volume control settings for the best listening level (BLL) of the children.

BEST LISTENING LEVELS

The most reliable method of finding BLLs involves speech audiometric procedures with each individual child. It is pertinent to remember, however, that even this technique has its limitations. For example, a considerable number of hearing-impaired children, because of degree of hearing loss, linguistic development, other handicaps, age or a combination of these factors may not be able to take part in speech audiometric testing. Furthermore, individual speech audiometric testing at various intensity levels and using a number of STUs, GHAs or both may prove too laborious and time consuming for a considerable number of teachers of the deaf.

Partly because of these limitations, several authors including Brooks (1973), Martin (1973), Morris (1975) and Powell and Tucker (1976) developed a number of formulae for calculating the optimum listening levels of hearing aid users. The formulae put forward are primarily based on pure tone hearing measurements and as such they exhibit significant deficiencies which have been well documented by Martin, Brooks and Morris (1977).

It needs to be noted, for example, that the optimum listening levels derived from some of these formulae were expressed in dB SPL and teachers and parents were advised to transfer these values directly on to the volume control settings of their respective STUs or GHAs. The implementation of this advice can lead to serious difficulties for (*a*) it cannot be assumed (without proper measurement) that a particular value in dB, say for example 125 dB as shown on the dial reading of a GHA or STU is identical in intensity to the 125 dB SPL as derived from the formulae (very few schools or units for hearing-impaired children have the necessary equipment and expertise to carry out the proper measurements); (*b*) formulae based on pure tone measurements do not take into consideration the wide differences existing in the acoustic properties of the speech of different teachers.

In view of these deficiencies, Markides (1980*c*) put forward a method for finding the BLLs of hearing-impaired children. This method has been widely used and has proved to be very quick and reliable and can be applied with the great majority of hearing-impaired children. It is independent of instrument variability and relates directly to the speech qualities of individual teachers. The method is as follows:

1 Find the uncomfortable listening level (ULL) of the child in each ear separately on your equipment, be it STU or GHA. Use the stimulus word 'go' and instruct the child on the following lines:

> I am going to say the word 'go' like this '. . . go . . . go . . . go . . .'. To start with I am going to say it very quietly, but gradually I am going to make it louder and louder and louder. Please listen carefully and tell me when it is too loud for you and you don't like it.

Reinforce these instructions with demonstration. When speaking the word 'go' into the microphone of the STU or GHA it is important

(*a*) to maintain a normal loudness level for speech;

(*b*) to adjust the gain control of the equipment so that the maximum excursion of the needle teachers 0 dB but does not penetrate into the red area of the VU meter; and

(*c*) to be as natural as possible and to avoid giving visual clues to the child pertaining to the loudness level generated.

The word 'go' is recommended for use in finding the ULL mainly because

(*a*) it is a relatively high intensity word, thus providing a safeguard against overamplification; and

(*b*) its frequency spectrum covers mainly the lower speech frequencies (most hearing-impaired children have better hearing at the lower speech frequencies than at the higher speech frequencies).

2 The BLLs of the child (for binaural listening) lie 5 to 15 dB (average 10 dB) immediately below the ULLs obtained.

3 For example:

(*a*) Right ear – ULL = 115 dB re: dial reading of amplification equipment used.
Left ear – ULL = 125 dB re: dial reading.

(*b*) Right ear – BLL = 115 − 10 = 105 dB (range 100 to 110 dB).
Left ear – BLL = 125 − 10 = 115 dB (range 110 to 120 dB).

4 Once the ULL in each ear is ascertained, try as first settings for BLL (binaural hearing) a combination of ULL − 5 dB in the left ear and ULL − 5 dB in the right ear. Converse with the child and if these settings are too loud decrease the intensity in one or both ears (as the case may be) in 5 dB steps until the child indicates that it is acceptable to him. The final acceptable levels for binaural hearing should be within the range already stated.

5 When the ULL of the child is beyond the maximum output of the equipment used, it is recommended to accept (in the first instance) the maximum acoustic output as the BLL of the child.

6 Note that the BLL of each child may fluctuate from day to day, especially when the child has a cold. The method suggested for finding the BLLs takes only 1 to 2 minutes per child to implement and therefore retests when necessary are advisable.

AUDITORY TRAINING

In 1939 Goldstein referred to auditory training as 'the stimulation or education of the hearing mechanism and its associate sense organs by sound vibration as applied either by voice or any sonorous instrument'. He included in this differentiation of pitch, rhythm, accent, volume and inflection as well as analysis and synthesis of speech sounds presented as tactile impressions. Wedenberg (1951) considered auditory training as 'a procedure directed at systematic and individual exploitation of the existing hearing with a certain suppression – but only stressed in the beginning – of the visual sense'. Carhart (1961) referred to it as 'the process of teaching the child or adult who is hard of hearing to take full advantage of sound cues which are still available to him'.

Several other authors avoided defining auditory training. Instead they stated major aims. For example, according to Hudgins (1954), the major aims of auditory training are the following:

(a) the development of auditory speech perception;
(b) better speech, which includes greater intelligibility, more natural voices and rhythmic speech;
(c) a broader and more flexible language development; and
(d) acceleration of the general education programme as a result of improved communication skills.

Watson (1964) identified five aims:
(a) greater understanding of the spoken language of others;
(b) more rapid development of the use of language by the child and its extension in the direction of normality;

(c) better speech by the child in terms of voice quality, articulation and rhythm;

(d) higher attainments in scholastic subjects, especially in basic skills, and

(e) better social and emotional adjustments through the provision of a direct link, however tenuous, with other people and the world at large.

Both Watson and Hudgins agree that for children the ultimate aim of auditory training is to maximise the amount of information they can extract primarily from the stimuli reaching them through the auditory channel.

Although most teachers of the deaf agree that a hearing-impaired person should be helped to use his residual hearing to the maximum there is disagreement as to whether auditory training should exist as a separate (re)habilitative procedure. Watson (1964) stated:

> The term auditory training will from henceforth be dropped since it implies a 'training of hearing'. Attempts through formal exercises either to improve hearing or to improve the use made of residual hearing, when they have focused attention on hearing alone have either failed or have just not justified the time and effort spent on them. It is therefore emphasised that this use of residual hearing is part of a multisensory approach . . . It is not a subject for which separate time needs to be set apart, except for some occasional short periods when listening is emphasised more than looking. If such a description of the use of residual hearing is accepted then it is evident that it will be used in the main as an adjunct to lipreading. It will, in fact, be exposure to sound, but it will be planned and systematically directed exposure with improvement in auditory perception as a possible by-product.

Contrary to this, Carhart (1961) advocated the use of specific auditory training procedures for the improvement of speech perception. He included in these procedures the differentiation between gross sounds, drill practice for discrimination between dissimilar speech sounds, and finally fine auditory discrimination between phonemes with similar acoustic structure.

While it is recognised that Watson's approach is a sensible one, it is felt that some hearing-impaired children will derive benefit from specialised and systematic auditory training as advocated by Carhart. The decision as to which method or combination of methods to adopt for each individual child must, in the final analysis, rest with the class teacher.

USE OF VISION

Ocular audition, labiomancy, labiology, lipreading, speechreading, visual hearing, visual listening and visual communication are all terms that have been used to describe a process by which a person ascribes meaning to speech that reaches him through the visual pathway. At present the most widely used terms are lipreading and speechreading and in this chapter both terms will be adopted and used interchangeably.

Lipreading is a complex task and it has traditionally formed an integral part of deaf education. Its ultimate aim is to maximise the amount of information that the hearing-impaired person can extract primarily from the speech stimuli reaching him through his visual modality.

The organs of speech that contribute most to visual reception of speech are the lips, the tongue and the degree of opening of the mouth. The various degrees of lip rounding, spreading and protrusion provide important cues. For example, in the production of /u/ as in 'boot' the lips are considerably rounded while in the production of /i/ as in 'seed' the lips are spread. Protrusion and lip rounding together help in the recognition of /tʃ/ as in 'church' and /ʃ/ as in 'ship'. In the production of /p, b, m/ the lips are brought together and /f/ and /v/ are characterised by a contact of the lower lip and the upper teeth. Observation of the tongue position facilitates the recognition of the consonant phonemes /θ, ð, l, t, d, n/. From observation of the degree of opening of the mouth together with visual information from other articulators we obtain cues important in the differentiation between vowels, e.g. between /a/ as in 'arm' and /ɪ/ as in 'sit'.

The suprasegmental or prosodic aspects of speech, such as loudness, pitch, intonation and duration are extremely difficult to identify through lipreading alone. The segmental aspects of speech, however, are more easily identifiable through lipreading. The main factors influencing their visual reception are (a) the degree of visibility of the movement and (b) the similarity of the visual characteristics of the articulatory movements between speech sounds.

DEGREE OF VISIBILITY

Speech sounds are produced by the movable organs of speech (vocal cords, soft palate, jaw, tongue and lips), which modify the air flow from the lungs. The production of each speech sound thus involves a distinctive combination of fine articulatory movements which may or may not be visually identifiable. The American Society for the Hard of Hearing (quoted by O'Neill, 1951) undertook a study into the relative visibility values of each speech sound and devised a method for calculating the visibility of any speech sample. Their results showed that the most difficult consonants for visual identification were /k, g, ŋ, h/ and the most easy /p, b, ʃ, z, tʃ, dʒ, f, v, θ, ð, m, j, w/. Vowels in general were found to be easier for visual identification than consonants, with the vowels /ɛ, ɪ, ɜ, ʊ, ʌ, ə/ being the most difficult and /a, æ, ɔ, ou, ʊ, ɔɪ, aʊ/ the most easy. The results of this study, however, have not been widely accepted (O'Neill, 1951) as the authors failed to take into consideration the effect of adjoining phonemes in rapid speech on the visual distinctiveness of individual phonemes. Similar studies by Heider and Heider (1940) and Watson (1956) can be criticised on the same grounds.

SIMILARITY OF VISIBLE ARTICULATORY MOVEMENTS

Speech sounds can be divided into two major groupings, vowels and consonants. The visual characteristics of each group will be dealt with separately. Acoustically each speech sound, be it vowel or consonant, is unique in structure; visually this is not true, however. Many speech sounds have *identical visual articulatory movements* and such sounds are referred to as *homophenes*. This term must not be confused with the similar term *homophones* which refers to speech symbols that have the same sound as others.

Vowels

Theoretically, each of the vowels is visually distinctive. In practice, that is in running speech, their distinctive visibility is clouded by adjacent sounds. Although this point has been made by Nitchie (1912), Kinzie and Kinzie (1931) and by Ewing (1941) it is often ignored in speechreading instruction. Woodward and Lowell (1964), Berger (1970), and Berger, de Pompei and Droder (1970) produced experimental evidence which showed conclusively that none of the vowels can be visually identified correctly under conditions of pure lipreading. Fisher (1968) suggested that vowels form only four groups of homophenes and not twelve groups hitherto accepted in traditional classification. Fisher's grouping was as follows:

1   i, ɪ, ɔɪ, əɪ
2   e, ɛ, ʌ, ɜ, aɪ
3   æ, a, aʊ
4   ɔ, a, ʊ, u

O'Neill (1954) found that vision alone contributed 29·5 per cent to the recognition of vowels while Woodward and Lowell (1964) and Berger (1972) reported correct visual identification of vowels averaging 49 per cent and 53·1 per cent respectively. These figures are below acceptable performance (60–70%, Ewing 1941) for effective day-to-day communication.

Consonants

Consonants can be classified according to their place of production, their manner of production, and whether they are voiced, unvoiced or nasalised. Their classification, however, is modified considerably in rapid conversational speech. Although acoustically voiced/unvoiced features and nasalisation of consonants can be easily distinguished, visually it is very difficult to do so (Larr, 1959). Most of the workers in this field (Bruhn, 1942; Burchett, 1950; Clegg, 1953; Ewing, 1967) accept that there are the following twelve categories of consonant homophenes:

1	p, b, m	7	l
2	f, v	8	s, z
3	w	9	ʃ, ʒ, tʃ, dʒ
4	r	10	j
5	θ, ð	11	k, g, ŋ
6	t, d, n	12	h

This classification is mainly based on the point of contact of articulation. Woodward and Lowell (1964) challenged the above traditional classification of consonant homophenes and suggested that there are only the following four consonant homophenous groups:

1 p, b, m
2 f, v
3 w, r
4 θ, ð, t, d, n, l, s, z, ʃ, tʃ, dʒ, j, k, g, ŋ, h

Fisher (1968) provided additional evidence against the traditional classification of the visual distinctiveness of consonants on five homophenous groupings:

1 p, b, m, d
2 f, v
3 w, r
4 t, d, n, ŋ, s, z, ʃ, j, h
5 k, g

For the final position he found the following consonant homophenes:

1 p, b
2 f, v
3 θ, ð, t, d, n, l, s, z
4 ʃ, ʒ, dʒ, tʃ
5 k, g, m

Berger (1972) reported that the traditional classification of consonants is essentially correct.

The cumulative writings of these authors show that correct identification of consonants through vision ranges from 30 to 40 per cent for initial consonants and only 20 to 30 per cent for final consonants. According to Ewing (1941) a discrimination of 70 per cent for consonants is required for effective understanding of speech. Clearly this cannot be achieved through vision alone.

Words

In addition to homophenous phonemes, the English language consists of a high proportion of homophenous words. There are also words that sound the same (homophones) which a listener can only differentiate through context. Words such as 'bear'/'bare', 'two'/'too' and 'bad'/ 'mat'/'pat'/'pan' are quite common in the English language and they tend to create speechreading difficulties and sometimes they can elicit embarrassing responses. Several authors have attempted to quantify the frequency distribution of homophenous words in the English language but their calculations are mainly based on experience rather than experimentation.

Nitchie (1915) stated that about 50 per cent of the words in the English language are homophenous to one or more other words. Kinzie and Kinzie (1931) and Bruhn (1949) stated that 50 per cent of all speech elements are invisible or indistinguishable while Wood and Blakely (1953) put this down to 11–17 per cent. According to Vernon and Mindel (1971) and Berger (1972) 40–60 per cent of the words of the English language are homophenous. It can be concluded that whatever the actual proportion of homophenous words in the English language, they are basically detrimental to speechreading accuracy.

It has been found by Taaffe and Wong (1957) that word length affects lipreading performance with two-letter words being more difficult to speech read than three-letter words. Similarly, Erber (1971) found significant improvements in lipreading of spondee words as compared to monosyllables. On the contrary, Brannon (1961) did not find significant differences in speechreading difficulty between monosyllables and spon-dees but reported improvement in speechreading of spondees presented in a sentence. The same results were reported by Sarrail in1951. Franks and Oyer (1967) found that familiar words are more easy to speechread than unfamiliar words and this was supported by Berger (1972) who stated that three-syllable words of the familiar type were the easiest words to speechread.

Sentences

Morris in 1944 (quoted by O'Neill and Oyer, 1961) investigated the effects of three aspects of stimulus materials upon speechreading performance: (a) the position of a sentence within a group of sentences, (b) the length of sentence and (c) the position of a group of sentences within a sequence of sentence groups. She reported a definite decline in speechreading scores as the length of the sentences increased but the 'speechreadability' of a sentence was not unduly influenced by its position within a group of sentences. Also she noted that a word was harder to speechread when placed in a long sentence than when placed in a shorter sentence. Essentially similar results were reported by O'Neill in 1954, Taaffe and Wong in 1957 and Schwartz and Black in 1967. These workers found phrases to be easier to speechread than sentences. Declarative sentences were found to be more difficult to lipread than interrogative or negative sentences.

THE LIPREADING TASK

In spite of the poverty of information on speech received through the visual modality, a lipreader, with good linguistic knowledge and an understanding of the contextual situation, can usually complete the partial message he receives through lipreading alone. Additional clues available to the lipreader include those stimuli that are directly related to the general background in which communication between two individuals is taking place and also to personal attributes of the speaker such as body posture and body movement, including gestures, age, sex, dress, ongoing activity and facial expressions.* For example, we attach meaning to gestures such as nodding of the head, a protruding tongue, a raised hand in a classroom; we can predict the utterance of a person trying to lift a heavy object; we receive clues from a person's facial expression – anger, pleasure, uncertainty, pain. On the basis of our observations we assign a role to the speaker especially when he wears a recognisable uniform or is engaged in a particular activity. The interpretation of these clues helps to clarify the verbal message. The most helpful additional clues are, of course, those provided by the use of residual hearing.

Other major factors that have been found to influence the lipreading process relate to the speaker (the visibility of the speaker, the rate of his speech, the amount of lip movement, the familiarity of the speaker, the sex of the speaker), the lipreader (visual acuity, attention, attitude and motivation, age, hearing loss, sex), and the environment (distance, lighting, distractions). For a full discussion of these factors refer to Markides (1977, 1980d).

Some teachers of the deaf discourage lipreading, especially during the formative years, because they believe that lipreading interferes with the development of the auditory reception of speech (Pollack, 1964). Others tend to teach lipreading intensively with particular emphasis on both phoneme and word recognition. The Ewings (1964) considered the first

---

* 'There's language in her eye, her cheek, her lip, Nay, her foot speaks.' *Troilus and Cressida*, IV. v. 54, Shakespeare.

practice as unrealistic and capricious and Ling (1976) was of the opinion that the second practice, because of its analytical nature, impedes rather than promotes speech communication. There is no doubt that lipreading, even for normally hearing people especially when trying to discriminate speech in adverse acoustic conditions, enhances speech reception and therefore it is of utmost importance to encourage the hearing-impaired child to look for visual clues in a speech communication process.

Both linguistic and speech development positively influence lipreading ability. In the first instance the child uses contextual clues more efficiently and in the second instance the child by referring to his own articulation movements can, to a certain extent, clarify the articulatory intentions of the speaker (Myklebust, 1960).

USE OF AUDITION AND VISION: AUDIO-VISUAL PROCESS

Although there are still differences of opinion over the advisability of combining hearing with vision with regard to the early education of hearing-impaired children there is no doubt that at present most teachers of the deaf, through experience and practice, support the combined use of audition and vision. Also the large number of experimental studies in the auditory–visual reception of speech that have been carried out with both normally hearing and hearing-impaired people support the audio-visual approach.

Laboratory studies with normally hearing people (Miller, Heise and Lichten, 1951; O'Neill, 1954; Erber, 1971; Sanders, 1971) have revealed more substantial improvement in speech reception when combining audition and vision than when employing either vision or audition alone. This improvement was evident especially with increasing unfavourable signal-to-noise ratio.

The auditory–visual speech reception abilities of hearing-impaired people have been studied both under laboratory conditions and in clinics. A plethora of researchers (Albright, 1944; Numbers and Hudgins, 1948; Hopkins, 1953; Prall, 1957; Evans, 1960, 1965; van Uden, 1960, 1970; Overbeck, 1960; Ewing, 1967; Duffy, 1967; Erber, 1971) showed that when the subjects both look and listen their speech reception is better than when they look alone or listen alone, sometimes by as much as 40 to 50 per cent (Hutton, 1959; McCormick, 1980).

USE OF VIBROTACTION

It is well documented that vibrotactile stimulation has been used by generations of teachers of the deaf in their attempts to develop and improve speech intelligibility. Both Braidwood and de l'Epée encouraged their children to see and to feel the articulatory movements of speech. Similar recommendations were put forward by Story (1915), Haycock (1933), Goldstein (1939) and more recently by the Ewings (1954).

Vibrotactile stimulation provides important clues relating to the perception of several suprasegmental aspects of speech such as loudness and duration. Vibrotactile stimulation plus kinaesthetic information derived from jaw and lip movement can help a hearing-impaired child to differentiate between vowels.

The voiced–voiceless distinction between consonants can easily be demonstrated through vibrotactile stimulation. The vibration of the nasal consonants /m, n, ŋ/ can be felt on the side of the nose. The sudden air flow associated with the onset of plosives /p, t, k/ can be felt on the muscles of the larynx. The differing breath streams associated with the production of /s/ and /ʃ/, concentrated and narrow for the first and more spread for the second, can be detected on the fingertips.

Vibrotactile stimulation has consistently been used to augment lipreading. One of the first workers to study speech perception among deaf people when using lipreading and vibrotactile stimulation was Gault (1926, 1927, 1928). He reported improvement in speech reception varying from 12 to 17 per cent when deaf people were given vibrotactile stimulation in addition to lipreading. Similar results were also reported by Pickett (1963) and Boothroyd (1972).

USE OF OTHER SYSTEMS

Several other systems have been developed to facilitate the speech reception and speech production of hearing-impaired children. Broadly speaking they can be divided into four categories: verbal instructions, cue systems, phonetic symbolisation systems and instrumental aids.

VERBAL INSTRUCTIONS

Teachers of the deaf often provide a variety of verbal instructions to help the children in correcting and monitoring their speech. These instructions vary from the general such as 'Use your voice', to the very specific 'You forgot the /s/ sound in "yes"'. Other common instructions include: 'Speak a little bit quicker, like this . . .'; 'Give me a good voice'; 'You left out the word "in" . . . in the road'. The Ewings (1954) advocated the early introduction and stabilisation of a specific vocabulary of words that will help a hearing-impaired child to acquire speech skills. For example, they suggested the teaching of the meaning of words *loud, very loud, quiet, very very quiet* with reference to the teaching of the control of loudness; *high* and *low* with reference to the teaching of pitch control; and *round, oval, hollow, press hard, press lightly, flick, flow, at the front, at the back, a little further back, a little further forward, put them together*, etc. with reference to the teaching of articulation and coarticulation of consonants and vowels. Verbal instructions based on these words can be very helpful in speech teaching provided, of course, the children understand the meaning of these words and relate such meaning to the movements and positions of their speech organs.

CUE SYSTEMS

A wide variety of cue systems have evolved specifically to help the hearing-impaired child in both speech reception and speech production. They will be presented here under a very loose categorisation consisting of (*a*) repetition, (*b*) exaggeration, (*c*) visual feedback, (*d*) gestural prompting, and (*e*) models, pictures and schemata.

Repetition

Environmental and situational factors such as background noise, reverberation, visual or acoustic distractions and inattention can affect the child's perception of his teacher's speech or his own speech or both. In these instances simple repetition may be sufficient to elicit the correct response.

Exaggeration

Hearing-impaired children, because of their auditory limitations or because of hearing aid distortion or both, may not be able to perceive a clear acoustic image of a word, a phrase, or a sentence when spoken in a natural manner. For example, the child may not be able to perceive the three syllables in the word 'potatoes' or he may not be able to differentiate the syllables in terms of stress. The teacher may attempt correction by exaggerating syllable duration or syllable intensity and by reinforcing this exaggeration with gestural cueing in the form of tapping or clapping. Exaggeration is also used in correcting articulation, in inserting missing words and in a wide variety of other situations. For example, when the child misses the final consonant /s/ as in 'yes' or misses the article 'the' in the phrase 'on the tree' the teacher may try to correct these mistakes by exaggerating the production of the missing speech elements – 'yeSSS', 'on . . . THE . . . tree'.

A word of caution is required here. Exaggeration distorts speech and if used extensively can bring about the opposite results from those intended. Whenever exaggeration or intentional distortion is used by the teacher the correct pattern of production must follow immediately.

Visual feedback

This refers primarily to the use of a mirror in the speech teaching process. Both the teacher and the child sit in front of the mirror and the child is asked to observe carefully the speech movements of the teacher and then to try and imitate them. Bell (1916) and the Ewings (1954) recommended the use of mirrors but Haycock (1933) and more recently Ling (1976) were not very keen on this. The present author has not found it necessary to use a mirror in a speech teaching situation except on one or two occasions when some action needed to be taken in order to avoid the unintentional projectiles of saliva emanating from the child's mouth!

Visual cues provided by simple objects such as a piece of paper or cotton, or anything else that moves as a result of slight air pressure, can be useful in demonstrating the production of certain sounds. For example, the plosion involved in the production of the consonant /p/ can be easily demonstrated with a piece of paper on the back of the hand. This approach, although practical in nature, can lead to incorrect articulatory movements by exaggerating the amount of breath required in producing a particular sound.

Colours have also been used to differentiate certain aspects of speech. For example, blue for unvoiced sounds, red for voiced and brown for nasals. This development has not been found practical although, according to Pickett (1981), in Japan a colour TV receiver is being used experimentally as a speech trainer. The three colour channels of the TV are used to represent the voiced aspect of speech, that is vowels and semi-vowels. These speech features vary with the vocal tract shape and thus the colour indications may be useful for teaching the correct movements of the vocal tract.

Gestural prompting

Gestures may be used to draw the child's attention to acoustic events relating to pitch change, loudness change, pause, stress, rate of speaking or intonation, or to certain aspects of speech such as voicing, nasality, plosion or friction. For example, a finger touching the side of the nose indicates nasality, a quick sweep of the hand indicates an increase in the rate of speaking, a hand on the chest indicates voicing, a raising of the hand indicates an increase in loudness. Gestural promptings emphasise speech but they need to be discarded as soon as they have served their purpose.

Models, pictures and schemata

Life-size models of the speech organs, usually a cross-section of the head, are sometimes used to explain and demonstrate the positioning of the different speech organs, especially the tongue, in the production of phonemes. These demonstrations are sometimes reinforced with pictures and schematic representations and they are directed mainly to older deaf children who have the necessary knowledge and background to conceptualise and abstract the necessary information.

The Ewings (1954) suggested the use of hand analogies to demonstrate certain articulatory movements. They used one hand to represent the roof of the mouth and the other hand to represent the tongue and its movements. For the production of /t/ and /d/ for example, the child is asked to flick the tip of his tongue at the front and for the production of /k/ and /g/ the child is asked to flick at the back. In the first instance the child is shown the index finger flicking at the front of the hand representing the palate and in the second instance the index finger flicks at the back of the hand. For those children who have been taught speech by the Ewings' method, hand analogies may be meaningful but for other children they cannot be anything else but confusing.

PHONETIC SYMBOLISATION SYSTEMS

These systems can be divided into two categories: manual methods and grapheme symbols.

Manual methods
Manual methods include mainly finger-spelling and signing, the Danish Mouth–Hand system, and Cornett's Cued Speech.

Finger-spelling refers to the spelling out of the word, letter by letter on the fingers. It can be done either with one hand or with both hands. Signing may follow the grammatical and syntactical sequence of a language or it may concentrate only on key words and phrases. In view of the obvious differences between manual modes of communication and speaking, it is highly unlikely that a hearing-impaired child can synchronise the information from each one of these modes and attend to them simultaneously. In addition to this, both finger-spelling and signing interfere with the temporal aspects of speech, thus hindering rather than promoting good speech intelligibility.

The Danish Mouth–Hand system was invented and published in 1902 by George Forchhammer, a Danish teacher of the deaf. The system consists of a systematic set of hand positions to indicate the invisible speech phonemes to the hearing-impaired person. It is widely used in Denmark in the rehabilitation of deafened adults. Users of this system testify to its effectiveness but there is very little experimental work to substantiate these claims. Deafened adults tend to speak abnormally slowly when using this system and this, in the long run, may have adverse effects on the intelligibility of their speech. As far as the writer knows this system has not been used in the education of English-speaking children.

Cornett's Cued Speech system is intended as a supplement to lipreading

(Cornett, 1964). Its basic rationale is similar to that of the Danish Mouth–Hand system. It uses hand configurations to help the lipreader identify those speech phonemes that are particularly difficult to recognise from lip movements alone. This system is not widely used in the United Kingdom. Its long-term contribution to speech development has not yet been evaluated.

Grapheme symbols

These systems use the written form to represent sounds. During the last hundred years several systems, such as A. M. Bell's Visible Speech (Bell, 1872), van Praagh's Pictorial Key Word system (van Praagh, 1884), the Northampton Charts (Worcester, 1915) and more recently the Initial Teaching Alphabet (Pitman, 1962), have been developed or suggested as possible aids to speech development. With the exception of the Northampton Charts none of the other systems has stood the test of time. Although the Northampton Charts are still widely used in the USA their popularity is declining and it is of significance to note that they have been virtually ignored on this side of the Atlantic.

Writing, based on traditional orthography, is widely used as an aid to speech teaching especially with older children who have acquired reading skills. It is used mainly to supplement oral speech by emphasising missing words or phonemes. It is also used (a) to show continuity of articulation and breath groups by grouping words together, (b) to show syllable or word stress by using stress signs, and (c) to show speech rhythm by using the necessary intonational contours or markings. Care must be taken, however, to see that the act of reading does not interfere with the spontaneity, fluency and quality of speech.

INSTRUMENTAL AIDS

Several attempts have been made to develop electronic speechreading aids. These attempts were initiated mainly in the USA and as yet the resulting devices are not widely used.

Upton (1968) developed one of the first electronic speechreading aids. The lipreader wears eyeglasses on which five small lights are used as indicators to differentiate between voiced, fricative and stop speech features. Upton has reported only limited success with this device especially when it was used in noisy environments.

Upton's device was later on modified and developed in collaboration with Pickett (1977) at Gallaudet College, USA. The new equipment that emerged indicates the following speech features as difficult to speechread: high frequency friction (s-sound), low frequency friction (sh-sound), stops, and the low frequency murmur of nasal consonants. Initial results with this equipment showed only a 7 per cent improvement over speechreading alone. The usefulness of this aid is totally negated in noisy situations.

The Central Institute of the Deaf in the USA developed and tested a tactual lipreading aid. It employs a larynx microphone, a speech microphone and a noise microphone. The signals from these microphones are fed to three vibrators which are attached to the fingers of the speechreader. Initial results with this device revealed improvement in speech reception varying from 7 to 18 per cent over speechreading alone. This is a cumbersome piece of equipment which again is greatly affected by background noise.

Recently, several attempts have been made in the United Kingdom (Douek, Fourcin, Moore and Clarke, 1977), Australia (Tong, Clark, Seligman and Patrick, 1980), Denmark, and the USA (Levitt, Pickett and Houde, 1980; McPherson and Davis, 1978) to augment speech reception among very severely deaf people by using 'electrical hearing', also referred to as 'cochlear implants'. These tiny implanted electrodes can stimulate directly the auditory nerve and it has been claimed that they enhance lipreading ability sometimes by as much as 54 percentage points. Work in this area is currently being pursued with vigour in several centres around the world, but the effectiveness of these developments awaits confirmation.

In the last few decades a considerable amount of time and effort has been devoted to the development of a wide variety of electronic speech training aids. These developments have ranged from simple devices such as the 'S' indicator, the voiced–voiceless indicator and the nasality indicator, to more complex systems such as the artificial palate, the laryngograph (Abberton, Parker and Fourcin, 1977) and, of course, spectrographic display (Strong, 1975).

Other recent developments relate to artificial speech and speech recognition systems. They are based on highly sophisticated computing techniques and their *modus operandi* is as follows. Deaf persons with very poor speech intelligibility type their message into a synthesiser which responds orally; their normally hearing correspondents reply, speaking into a central speech recogniser which then sends a written version of the spoken message to the teletype of the deaf person. At present there are commercial portable speech synthesisers, such as the HandiVoice, but their use among deaf people is very rare.

Results achieved through the use of these devices in terms of speech improvements have been generally disappointing. The few relevant studies in this area have failed to show any significant improvement in speech skills associated with the use of such specialised aids (Boothroyd, 1973; Stratton, 1974; Houde, 1980). Note also that none of these aids has come into widespread teaching use. It may be that, with further developments, this situation will change but at present it seems that the benefits provided may not justify the additional expenditure and effort involved in their use.

SUMMARY

A hearing impairment in childhood interferes with normal speech development and in view of this the hearing-impaired child requires specialised help to acquire, develop and maintain good intelligible speech. The use of residual hearing in the acquisition and development of speech skills by hearing-impaired children is important. Relevant information on the use of amplification and on the optimum listening conditions required for maximum benefit has been presented and discussed.

It must be stressed that all hearing-impaired children supplement their auditory speech information with additional cues which they extract from the speech reaching them through the visual modality, that is, lipreading. The use of vibrotaction has been discussed, as have the uses of a wide variety of other aids to speech reception and speech production.

The cumulative evidence emerging from this strongly supports a multisensory approach in the teaching of speech to hearing-impaired children with audio-vision, supplemented when necessary by vibrotactile stimulation, being the most effective combination of sensory modes for speech reception and speech production.

CHAPTER TEN

The delivery system: Principles, objectives and strategies

In foregoing chapters the emphasis has been on the speech of hearing-impaired children. This chapter will concentrate on several important aspects of the speech delivery system – on the main principles, objectives and strategies employed in the teaching of speech to hearing-impaired children and on the key professional responsible for speech development, namely the teacher of the deaf.

PRINCIPLES

The preceding chapters in this section presented and discussed the scientific base of speech reception and speech production with special reference to the hearing-impaired child. The core of information presented is hereby summarised in a series of broad principles onto which effective speech teaching strategies can be based.

1 Speech is learned, not instinctive, and as such it can be taught to the great majority of hearing-impaired children. Note that it is acknowledged within this principle that a number of hearing-impaired children, because of degree of hearing loss, pathology of deafness, additional handicaps, or a combination of factors are unable to develop functional speech skills.
2 Speech is learned best through audition and therefore maximum use of residual hearing is required.
3 The use of vision always enhances the auditory speech perceptual process. Therefore the hearing-impaired child should be encouraged to use both audition and vision (the audio-visual approach) in a speech training process. This can also be supplemented by the use of vibrotaction when necessary.
4 Speech in the normally hearing child develops in an orderly manner

following well documented, logical and interrelated stages. The hearing-impaired child needs to go through the same pattern of development but to do so he may require expert help and guidance and certainly a much longer period of time.

5 The normally hearing child develops speech skills primarily as a result of continual auditory stimulation, incessant exposure to speech, unceasing encouragement and hours and hours of practice. This is equally true for hearing-impaired children, but they, because of their handicap, may also require specialised instruction in order to develop, improve and maintain acceptable speech skills.

6 Each hearing-impaired child has unique speech requirements, therefore individual speech training and remediation is essential. In this context regular individual speech assessment is required in order (a) to determine strengths and weaknesses, (b) to identify speech problems, and (c) to monitor progress.

7 Positive attitudes towards the value of oral communication encourage success in speech skills.

8 Success in speech development depends primarily on the parents, on the teacher of the deaf and on the educational establishment attended by the child. Parents need to be informed, cooperative and supportive. Teachers need (a) to believe that hearing-impaired children can develop intelligible speech, and (b) to have the necessary training and skills to teach speech. The educational establishment needs to foster an atmosphere that encourages speech within the school and an ethos that is relaxed yet demanding when it comes to the use of speech.

OBJECTIVES

The ultimate objective of speech training is to help the hearing-impaired child to develop, improve, maintain and use oral communication to exchange ideas, information and feelings with regard to his educational, social and leisure activities. In other words to develop speech skills and use them as a way of life.

In the process of achieving the long-term objective, the hearing-impaired child may require specialised help to master a series of interrelated speech skills which can be seen as a number of specific objectives or goals in speech training. Some of these specific objectives are as follows:

1 To vocalise and use voice meaningfully.
2 To develop a pleasant voice quality.
3 To develop good breath control.

4 To develop the suprasegmental aspects of speech, such as pitch, loudness, duration and rhythm.
5 To articulate correctly the phonemes of his native language, emphasising coarticulation and automaticity.
6 To put words together to form sentences and to articulate them using proper rhythm, accent, intonation and phrasing.
7 To associate speech with meaning and conceptual thinking.
8 To develop a positive attitude towards speaking and to use speech spontaneously.
9 To internalise and use spontaneously the speech skills mastered.
10 To develop appropriate strategies in dealing with difficult oral communication problems.
11 To develop, as far as possible, a self-monitoring audio visual and kinaesthetic feedback system for speech reception and speech production.

These are only a limited number of specific objectives in speech training. Many more can be quoted. It must not be assumed, however, that all these specific speech goals can be achieved within a relatively short period of time. Of course some of them will be but others are ongoing and require attention throughout the child's schooling and beyond. It is essential to remember that concentration on any one or any group of these specific objectives must not be allowed to divert attention from the ultimate goal. Undue emphasis on specifics interferes with the perception of the whole!

STRATEGIES

No attempt will be made here to give a detailed step-by-step description of speech teaching methodologies. This is beyond the scope of this book and it has already been done most ably and comprehensively by previous writers such as Haycock (1933), the Ewings (1954), Calvert and Silverman (1975) and Ling (1976).

Strategies in speech training are many and varied and those that suit one particular child may be inappropriate to another. This is because each hearing-impaired child is an individual with unique abilities and aptitudes and with unique auditory potential, personality and background. These factors affect the child's rate and style of learning and of necessity to meet individual needs, the teacher of the deaf has to be eclectic, versatile and flexible in her methods of teaching speech – a rigid and monolithic approach cannot satisfy the needs of all the children.

It is more appropriate therefore to concentrate on the principles and objectives already stated and leave the initiation, development, modification and implementation of speech teaching strategies to the class teacher provided, of course, that such a teacher has the necessary professional qualifications and expertise to do so. Within any speech training model or programme there is a plethora of strategies to be followed by the teacher and also there is a plethora of interrelated speech skills and sub-skills to be mastered by the children. It is only the class teacher, who knows the children best, who can choose the right teaching strategies to meet the learning needs of each individual child in his or her class.

Having said this, however, it is accepted that the class teacher requires some guidelines, in this case a speech training model, within which he or she can plan and operate. Not only does a speech training model provide continuity of approach but also brings about uniformity of purpose within an educational establishment. The speech training model recommended, based on the principles already stated and encompassing the objectives enumerated previously, is shown in Figure 10.1. It represents the teaching of speech at three interlocking levels – meaning, prosody, articulation – which in turn affect speech fluency and in the final analysis determine the degree of speech intelligibility.

Meaning in this context refers to language development (lexical, morphological, syntactic and semantic development) and conceptual thought. Prosody refers to voice quality, breath control, pausing, phrasing, stress, emphasis, intonation, rate of speaking, etc. Articulation

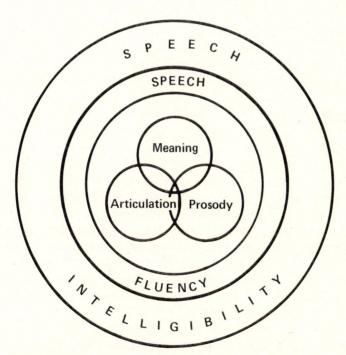

FIGURE 10.1 Outline of speech training model

refers to vocalisation, vowel production, diphthong production, consonant production, coarticulation of phonemes, words, phrases and sentences.

Most hearing-impaired children require training in all three levels with the emphasis of training shifting from one level to another depending on the stage of development and needs of the child. The interlocking nature of the three levels ensures, to a certain extent, that improvement in one carries over to the others. It needs to be pointed out, however, that undue emphasis of training in one or two of these levels, to the exclusion of the other(s), may actually interfere with rather than promote good intelligible speech. For example, speech teaching that emphasises solely the durational aspects of speech, to the exclusion of articulatory work, has very little to recommend it.

There are many speech skills and sub-skills to be mastered in each of the levels. For example, a particular hearing-impaired child may require intensive help with vocabulary development and use of language whilst another child's needs may be centred on the articulation of a particular phoneme, or on voice quality. The danger exists that the teacher in her endeavour to improve one specific speech sub-skill, such as articulation of final /s/, may, by putting too much emphasis on it, obscure the final objective of her teaching which is the development of fluent and intelligible speech. This danger can be avoided if speech sub-skills are always introduced and taught within the context of continuous speech and never in isolation. Of course, there will be instances where a particular speech sub-skill may need treatment in isolation before being injected back into continuous speech. This is an acceptable procedure provided the particular sub-skill being taught is immediately incorporated and practised in continuous and fluent speech.

The identification of speech skills and sub-skills to be taught is the domain of the teacher of the deaf. Identification is achieved through careful and ongoing assessment and this is an integral part of the speech training model recommended.

A multisensory approach to the teaching of speech, emphasising the audio-visual mode of speech reception, is recommended. Some hearing-impaired children may, of course, come to rely more on audition than vision and vice versa whilst others may require additional help from vibrotactile stimulation, speechreading and from specialised instrumental systems such as the laryngograph or the simple 'S' indicator. When children acquire competency in reading then a combination of audition, vision and the written form becomes a powerful avenue for speech acquisition and improvement.

Before any speech training occurs, however, a speech sample must be elicited from the child. This can happen spontaneously when the child simply wants to tell or ask about something or the teacher can stimulate the child to speak about a picture or a small activity or something else. When the teacher elicits the speech the situation is controlled but the child may not be interested. When the child utters speech spontaneously, internally generated ideas are being expressed, the situation is more meaningful and the child is more receptive to tuition. However, speech teaching must be carefully applied in such cases so that it does not disrupt the communication process. It is the writer's opinion that the conversational approach offers the best avenue for speech elicitation and correction. The teacher engages the child in conversation on topics, activities and interests that are meaningful to the child and the speech elicited is improved both in content and in clarity but, as stated previously, this must be achieved without any major dislocation of the flow of conversation.

The individual nature of speech teaching has been consistently emphasised in this book. What needs to be added here is that most hearing-impaired children require such individual attention on a daily basis with at least one 10 to 15 minute lesson per day.

Individual speech teaching can only succeed in an atmosphere that provides continuity of purpose and encourages and requires oral communication not only within the classroom but also outside in the playground, in the home and in the society at large. To achieve this it is essential to have cooperation between parents and teachers and also between teachers themselves.

THE TEACHER

Today's teacher of the deaf faces a very difficult task in that he or she needs to develop competencies and expertise in many and varied areas. Not only does a teacher of the deaf need to acquire theoretical and practical knowledge in a wide range of subjects, but also to abstract, synthesise and apply such knowledge to meet the individual needs of the children. Only capable and highly motivated teachers of the deaf can accomplish this task. Boothroyd (1980) was of the opinion that the profession of teaching the deaf in the USA seldom attracts such people. In the United Kingdom the situation is certainly different. On the whole the calibre of the people entering the profession in this country is high but perhaps on some courses training in the teaching of speech is not as intensive as it used to be twenty or thirty years ago.

There is a growing tendency among newly qualified teachers of the deaf, for example, to consider that the use of amplification alone plus exposure to normal patterns of speech is sufficient to meet the varied speech requirements of hearing-impaired children. This is certainly not so. Even with the use of the best amplifying equipment available and the best will in the world a considerable number of hearing-impaired children, because of severity of deafness, frequency resolution abnormalities or other complex speech perceptual problems, will never be able to receive and monitor speech through their auditory channel. In order to develop and maintain acceptable speech skills these children need to be taught speech using a multisensory approach on the lines of the methods and strategies used by previous generations of teachers of the deaf and so ably presented by authors such as Haycock (1933), the Ewings (1954), Calvert and Silverman (1975) and Ling (1976). It is no coincidence that speech therapists are increasingly being involved in the teaching of speech to hearing-impaired children. They are obviously better prepared than newly qualified teachers of the deaf to deal with the mechanical aspects of speech such as articulation and prosody. But this is precisely the danger. Their training may not have prepared them to deal with the development of speech and its function in verbal communication especially when both development and function are directly affected by deafness.

The basic issue arising from this relates to the selection and training of teachers of the deaf. Assuming that the right calibre of people have been selected (normally hearing, mature, interested, with acceptable educational standards, responsible, hard working, innovating, persevering, willing to learn) what then is the most appropriate training they need in order to emerge as competent and efficient speech teachers?

First, they need to develop special attitudes and techniques which foster, sustain and encourage the use of speech by the children.

Secondly, they require extensive knowledge in the following subject areas:

(a) normal speech development, speech physiology, speech reception and speech production, acoustics and phonetics;
(b) hearing impairment and its effects on these areas;
(c) the use of audition, vision, vibrotaction and their combinations in speech acquisition and development;
(d) the use of amplification equipment, visual and instrumental aids for speechteaching – their availability, advantages and limitations; and
(e) methods of developing, improving and evaluating the speech of hearing-impaired children.

Thirdly, they require practice under expert supervision in

(a) developing listening skills that will permit them to detect, identify and analyse speech problems (the Ewings (1954) referred to this as developing a 'discerning ear');
(b) giving speech lessons to hearing-impaired children representing a wide variety of speech problems and different levels of speech

competence (lessons need to be taken both on an individual basis and with small groups of children); and

(c) assessing and evaluating speech problems and planning remediation and help on a short- and on a long-term basis.

In the final analysis, however, success in speech teaching depends, to a large extent, on the support, guidance and advice the newly qualified teacher receives from the educational establishment in which he or she works. Course work can only lay the foundation: competence and efficiency come slowly through expert guidance, perseverance and practice.

SUMMARY

This chapter has put forward basic principles, objectives and strategies in the teaching of speech to hearing-impaired children. In particular it has developed and outlined a speech training model based on the principles and objectives stated, and dealt with the training and preparation of teachers of the deaf, especially with regard to the teaching of speech.

CONCLUDING REMARKS

There is no doubt that at present we possess an enormous amount of knowledge regarding the speech of hearing-impaired children. Also in the last two decades we have witnessed an unprecedented expansion of facilities in the relevant fields of education, medicine and audiology. We have considerable access to highly sophisticated electronic amplifying equipment. Our special educational system is rapidly becoming more flexible and more versatile in meeting individual needs. In spite of all this progress, however, there still remains a large number of hearing-impaired children who leave school without an acceptable degree of speech intelligibility. This state of affairs may be partly due to our delivery system – the speech teaching methods employed; the amount of speech teaching; the calibre of teaching; the interaction between teachers, pupils and parents; the speech environment prevailing in the school and, of course, the training, preparation and support of teachers of the deaf. It is the opinion of the writer that the number of hearing-impaired children leaving school with unintelligible speech can be greatly reduced if time, effort, research and application are focused on improving the delivery system. Of course, theoretical considerations concerning the teaching of speech must continue to develop but unfortunately in the last twenty years too much emphasis has been placed on theory and not enough on practice.

APPENDICES

Opposite: APPENDIX 1   Articulation test

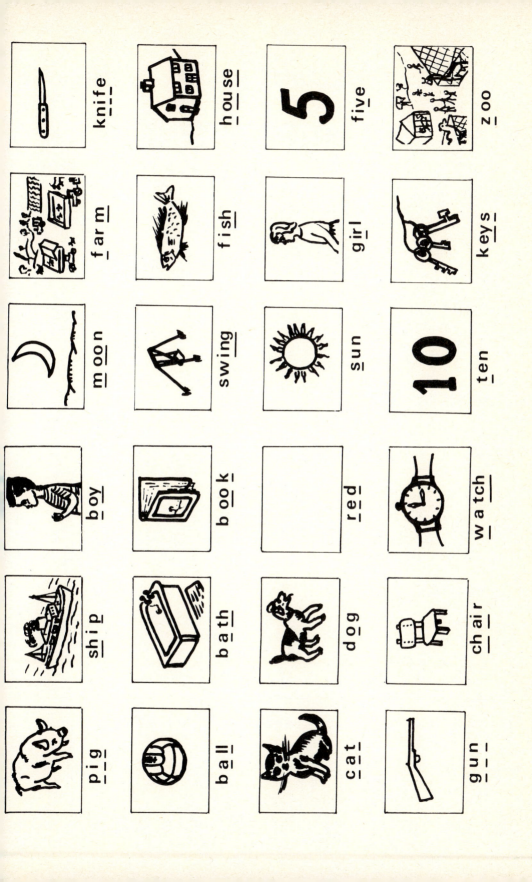

APPENDIX 2 Analysis of causes of deafness – all children in PHUs

% children

Age groups in years:	2	3	4	5	6	7	8	9	10	11	12	13	14	15	16	17	18	19	2–18
Number of children:	4	52	79	132	166	153	200	199	216	222	249	222	216	184	111	17	6	1	2429
CAUSES OF DEAFNESS																			
Prenatal																			
Heredity		9·6	6·3	9·1	10·2	7·8	5·5	10·1	6·5	7·2	6·4	5·9	8·8	5·4	6·3	11·8			7·4
Familial			2·5	1·5	4·8	5·2	5·5	3·5	5·6	4·5	6·8	4·1	3·2	2·7	2·7				4·2
Congenital			1·3	3·9	1·8	3·3	2·5	1·5	0·5	2·3	1·6	1·4	0·5	1·6	2·7				1·7
Genetic			3·8	0·8	1·2	3·3	2·5	2·5	0·9	1·8			0·5	1·1					1·2
Recessive			1·3		0·6														
Progressive			1·3		1·2									0·5	0·5				0·2
Chromosome abnormality																			
Osteogenesis imperfecta									0·5										
Syndromes:																			
Pierre Robin				0·8									0·5						
Waardenburg					0·6			0·5	0·9	0·9	0·8	0·5	0·5						0·2
Treacher Collins		1·9		1·5	1·2	1·3		0·5	0·9		0·8	0·9	0·5	0·5					0·7
Jervel, Lange-Nielsen							0·5												
Pendred																			
Klippel Feil																			
Turner																			
Crouzon																			
Down																			
External malformations		11·5		0·8	0·6		1·0	10·1	0·5	0·9			0·5	11·4					0·4
Maternal rubella		11·5	12·5	12·1	9·0	13·1	18·0	10·1	13·0	13·1	18·1	12·2	8·8	15·3	15·3	5·9			12·5
Cytomegalovirus					0·6										0·9				0·1
Toxaemia				0·8								0·5							0·1
Anaemia of pregnancy																			
Sickle cell anaemia																			
Drugs									0·5										
Perinatal																			
Anoxia		1·9	1·3	1·5	1·2	1·3	0·5	2·5	0·9	2·7	1·6	1·4	3·2	2·2	3·6	17·6			1·9
Birth injury		7·7	1·3	3·8	1·8	0·7	0·5	1·5		0·9		1·4	0·5	1·6	0·9				1·2

APPENDIX 2 (*cont.*)

Age groups in years:	2	3	4	5	6	7	8	9	10	11	12	13	14	15	16	17	18	19	2–18
Number of children:	4	52	79	132	166	153	200	199	216	222	249	222	216	184	111	17	6	1	2429
								% children											
Perinatal (*cont.*)																			
Prematurity		1·9	2·5	3·0		1·3	1·5	2·0	4·6	1·4	1·6	1·4	3·2	1·6	2·7				2·0
Kernicterus				0·8	0·6	2·0	3·0	1·5	2·4	1·0	1·2	1·4	1·9	3·3	2·7				1·7
Postnatal																			
Mastoidectomy													0·5	1·6	1·8				0·2
Ear operation (unsp.)																			
Chronic otitis media		5·8	1·3	0·8		2·0	0·5	0·5	0·9	0·9		1·4	3·2	2·2	0·9				1·1
Conductive (unsp.)			1·3	1·5		3·9	1·5	0·5	0·5	0·5	0·8	0·9	2·3	2·2	1·8				1·4
Measles, > 2 yrs age			1·3			0·7		0·5	0·5			0·5	0·5	1·1					0·3
Measles, < 2 yrs age					0·6		0·5	0·5		0·9	0·4	0·5	1·4		0·9				0·4
Meningitis, > 2 yrs age		7·7	3·8	2·3	1·2	2·0	2·5	3·0	3·2	4·1	1·6	1·4	1·4	2·2	1·8				2·3
Meningitis, < 2 yrs age		1·9	5·1	3·8	1·8	1·3	3·0	0·5	0·9		0·8	0·5	0·9	0·5	0·9				1·3
Mumps, > 2 yrs age												0·5							0·1
Mumps, < 2 yrs age				0·8		0·7		1·0			0·4	0·9	0·5	0·5					0·3
Whooping cough																			
Typhoid																			
Shingles																			
TB																			
Convulsions											0·4			0·5					
Virus (unsp.)					1·2	2·0	1·0			0·5			0·5	0·5	0·9	5·9			0·5
Measles vaccine		1·9	1·3																
Polio injection																			
Immunisation (unsp.)			1·3									0·5							0·1
Streptomycin				0·8				0·9				0·5	0·5						0·3
Steroids												0·5							
Concussion/Fractured skull			1·3								0·8	0·5	0·5	1·0					0·3
Scalding									0·5										
Unknown	48·1	59·5	59·5	50·0	59·0	48·4	50·5	54·8	54·6	56·8	55·8	61·3	55·1	54·3	53·2	58·8			54·9

APPENDIX 3   Analysis of causes of deafness – all children in schools for the deaf

Age groups in years:	2	3	4	5	6	7	8	9	10	11	12	13	14	15	16	17	18	19	2-19
Number of children:	7	35	31	68	104	137	135	162	216	251	304	336	345	351	194	36	29	2	2743
% children																			
CAUSES OF DEAFNESS																			
Prenatal																			
Heredity		20·0	19·4	13·2	11·5	7·3	3·7	6·2	7·4	5·2	5·3	5·1	7·8	6·0	5·2	11·1	6·9		6·7
Familial		2·9	9·7	2·9	2·9	6·6	3·0	2·5	2·8	5·6	5·3	3·0	5·5	2·8	4·1	11·1	13·8		4·3
Congenital		2·9	3·2	4·4	5·8	4·4	3·0	4·9	4·6	4·4	3·6	3·0	4·1	5·1	6·2				4·2
Genetic			3·2		1·0	1·5	1·5	0·6	1·4	0·4	0·7	0·3		0·6	0·5				0·6
Recessive																			
Progressive											0·3								
Chromosome abnormality																			
Osteogenesis imperfecta																			
Syndromes:																			
Pierre Robin					1·0				0·5										0·1
Waardenburg			3·2		1·9			0·6		0·4		0·6		1·0					0·4
Treacher Collins									0·5		0·3								0·1
Jervel, Lange-Nielsen									0·5										
Pendred																			
Klippel Feil			3·2							0·4		0·3							0·1
Turner												0·3							
Crouzon																			
Down																			
External malformations									0·5			0·6							0·1
Maternal rubella		5·7		13·2	10·6	19·7	22·2	11·7	16·2	19·9	22·4	22·9	18·8	21·4	19·1	25·0	24·1		19·2
Cytomegalovirus						0·7		0·6				0·3							
Toxaemia							0·7					0·3		0·9	1·0				0·3
Anaemia of pregnancy																			
Sickle cell anaemia											0·3								
Drugs											0·3								
Perinatal																			
Anoxia		2·9		1·5		1·5		1·9	2·3	0·4	1·6	1·8	2·3	0·6	1·5	2·8	10·3		1·6
Birth injury		5·7	3·2	2·9	1·0		0·7		0·9	0·8		0·6	1·7	0·9	1·5				0·9

APPENDIX 3 (*cont.*)

Age groups in years:	2	3	4	5	6	7	8	9	10	11	12	13	14	15	16	17	18	19	2–19
Number of children:	7	35	31	68	104	137	135	162	216	251	304	336	345	351	194	36	29	2	2743
									% children										
Perinatal (cont.)																			
Prematurity		2·9	3·2	5·9	1·9	0·7	2·2	2·5	1·4	0·8	2·0	1·5	3·5	3·4	1·5	2·8			2·3
Kernicterus		2·9			1·9	2·2	1·5	5·0	1·4	3·6	3·6	3·0	2·9	4·6	3·6	2·8			3·0
Postnatal																			
Mastoidectomy																			
Ear operation (unsp.)																			
Chronic otitis media					1·0				0·5					0·3	0·5				0·1
Conductive (unsp.)					1·0	0·7	0·7						0·3						0·1
Measles, >2 yrs age										0·8		0·3	0·3	0·3	1·5		3·4		0·3
Measles, <2 yrs age								0·6				0·3	0·3	0·6	1·0				0·3
Meningitis, >2 yrs age		5·7	3·2	1·5	1·0	2·9	1·5	3·1	3·2	4·0	3·3	3·3	2·0	3·1	1·0	5·6			2·8
Meningitis, <2 yrs age			6·5	4·4	2·9	2·9	3·0	4·9	5·6	6·0	3·9	4·2	2·9	1·7	5·2	2·8	6·9		3·9
Mumps, >2 yrs age						1·0						0·3	0·3						0·1
Mumps, <2 yrs age							0·7					0·3							0·1
Whooping cough					1·5					0·4		0·3	0·6						0·2
Typhoid																			
Shingles															0·5				
TB																			
Convulsions																			
Virus (unsp.)						1·9	0·7		1·2					0·6	0·5				0·3
Measles vaccine										0·4									
Polio injection																			
Immunisation (unsp.)									0·6		0·3			0·3	0·5				0·1
Streptomycin			3·2								0·3	1·2	0·3						0·3
Steroids											0·7								
Concussion/Fractured skull									0·5	0·4			0·3	0·3					0·1
Scalding																			
Unknown	48·6	48·6	38·7	47·1	51·9	47·4	53·3	52·5	49·5	45·0	45·7	46·4	45·5	45·6	42·8	36·1	34·5		46·6

APPENDIX 4 Analysis of additional handicap – all children in PHUs

Age groups in years:	2	3	4	5	6	7	8	9	10	11	12	13	14	15	16	17	18	19	2–18
Number of children:	4	52	79	132	166	153	200	199	216	222	249	222	216	184	111	17	6	–	2429
								% children											
ADDITIONAL HANDICAP																			
None		82·7	83·5	81·8	84·9	83·0	83·5	84·4	83·8	81·1	84·7	82·9	84·7	85·3	84·7	76·5			83·7
Aphasia			1·3						0·5		0·4		0·5		0·9				0·2
Asthma				0·8			1·0	1·5			0·4	0·5	0·9	0·5					0·5
Athetosis																			
Auditory sequencing abn.							0·5			0·5		0·5							0·1
Autistic														0·5					
Balance		1·9			1·2														0·1
Brain damage			2·5	1·8	3·0	2·0	1·0	0·5	0·5	0·5	1·2		1·0		0·9				0·9
Cleft palate		3·8		3·0	1·2	2·0	2·0	0·5		1·4	0·8	0·5	0·5	1·1					1·1
Diabetic																			
Diplegia																			
Disphasia									0·5	0·5									0·1
Dispraxia																			
Dyslexia																			
Ear sores, chronic																			
Elected mute			2·5		0·6														
Epilepsy						0·7	0·5	0·5		1·8	0·8		0·5	0·5	0·9				0·5
Heart condition						0·7	0·5	0·5	0·9	0·5	0·8	1·4	0·5		0·9				0·6
Hemiplegia										0·5			0·5						0·1
Hydroencephalic													0·5						
Hyperactivity							0·5	0·5		0·5	0·8	0·5							0·2
Language disorder			1·3	1·5		0·7	0·5	0·5	0·9	0·5									0·4
Learning difficulties							1·0		0·5		0·4								0·2
Lisping					0·6														0·1
Maladjustment (behaviour, social, emotional problems)				0·8		1·3	0·5	2·5	1·4	1·4	0·8	0·5	1·4	1·1		5·9			1·0

APPENDIX 4 (*cont.*)

% children

	2	3	4	5	6	7	8	9	10	11	12	13	14	15	16	17	18	19	2–18
Age groups in years:																			
Number of children:	4	52	79	132	166	153	200	199	216	222	249	222	216	184	111	17	6	–	2429
Low IQ/ESN				1·5	2·4	2·0	1·5	3·0	2·8	2·7	3·6	2·7	1·4	4·3	0·9	5·9			2·4
Mental handicap, severe		1·9		0·8				0·5			0·8	0·9							0·3
Microcephalic		1·9																	0·1
Monoplegia									0·5										
Motor control/poor coordination			1·3	3·1	1·2			1·0		1·4	0·8	0·5	0·5	0·5	1·8				0·7
Nasality, excessive											0·4	0·5			0·9				0·1
Pernicious anaemia													0·5						
Purpura													0·5						
Curvature of spine																			
Facial deformity				0·8		0·7			0·5			0·5	0·5	0·5					0·2
Limping												0·5	0·5						0·1
Malocclusion of jaws											0·4								
Rickets																			
Spina bifida		1·9		0·8		0·7		0·5					0·5		0·9				0·2
Weak/delicate			1·3							0·5			0·9		0·9				0·2
Unspecified (physical)		1·9				0·7				0·5	0·4	0·5		0·5	0·9				0·3
Spasticity		1·9	1·3			1·3	0·5		1·4	1·8	0·8		3·2	0·5	0·9	5·9			1·2
Short-term memory										0·5				0·5					
Stammer																			
Tongue-tied						0·7	0·5					0·5							
Thyroid deficiency																			
Visual problems		1·9	5·1	3·8	4·8	3·9	5·5	3·5	5·1	4·1	1·6	5·0	2·3	2·7	3·6	5·9			3·8
Blind (total)																			
Colour blind															0·9				
Retinitis pigmentosa																			
Unspecified																			

APPENDIX 5   Analysis of additional handicap – all children in schools for the deaf

% children

Age groups in years:	2	3	4	5	6	7	8	9	10	11	12	13	14	15	16	17	18	19	2–19
Number of children:	7	35	31	68	104	137	135	162	216	251	304	336	345	351	194	36	29	2	2743
ADDITIONAL HANDICAP																			
None	74·3	71·0		88·2	80·8	73·0	74·1	76·5	74·1	84·9	81·9	76·2	78·8	81·5	77·8	88·9	96·6		79·1
Aphasia													0·6	0·3					0·1
Athetosis						1·5						0·9			0·5				0·2
Auditory sequencing abn.							0·7												0·1
Autistic					1·0			0·6			0·3								0·1
Balance											0·3				0·5				0·1
Brain damage						2·2	1·4	1·9	0·5	0·3	0·3	0·9	0·3	0·3	0·5				0·6
Cleft palate		5·7			1·0	1·5		1·2	0·9			0·9	0·9	0·9					0·7
Diabetic											0·3								
Diplegia													0·6		0·5				
Disphasia																			
Dispraxia								0·6											
Dyslexia									0·5		0·3				0·5				0·1
Ear sores, chronic																			
Elected mute																			
Epilepsy				1·5						0·4		0·3	1·2	1·1					0·4
Heart condition						1·5	0·7	0·6		1·2	1·0	1·2	0·6	0·6					0·6
Hemiplegia											0·3	0·3	0·3	0·3					0·2
Hydroencephalic					1·0			1·9	0·5	0·4	1·0	0·3	0·3						0·5
Hyperactivity		2·9				2·2			0·9	0·4	0·7	0·6	0·6						0·4
Language disorder					1·0		0·7	1·2	0·5	0·4	0·7	0·6	0·6						0·5
Learning difficulties				1·5		1·5	2·2	0·6	3·2		0·3	0·9	0·3	0·3	0·5				0·7
Lisping						1·5										2·8			
Madadjustment (behaviour, social, emotional problems)				1·5	1·0	1·5	1·5		1·4	1·6	1·6	3·9	1·2	1·7	0·5				1·3

APPENDIX 5 (*cont.*)

% children

Age groups in years:	2	3	4	5	6	7	8	9	10	11	12	13	14	15	16	17	18	19	2–19
Number of children:	7	35	31	68	104	137	135	162	216	251	304	336	345	351	194	36	29	2	2743
Low IQ/ESN		2·9	3·2		5·8	4·4	6·7	3·1	4·6	4·8	3·0	3·6	4·3	4·0	5·2	5·6			4·0
Mental handicap, severe			3·2	2·9	2·9	0·7	0·7	2·5	3·7	1·2	0·3	0·6	0·6	0·9	1·0				1·3
Microencephalic						0·7			0·5		0·7								0·1
Monoplegia										0·4									
Motor control/poor coordination				1·5			0·7		1·4		0·3	1·2	0·9	0·6	0·5				0·6
Nasality, excessive																			
Pernicious anaemia							0·7	0·6											0·1
Purpura																			
Curvature of spine																			
Facial deformity									0·5			0·3							0·1
Limping												0·3							
Malocclusion of jaws																			
Rickets																			
Spina bifida					1·9						0·7				0·5				0·2
Weak/delicate			3·2										0·3	0·3	0·5				0·1
Unspecified (physical)						0·7	0·7	0·6		0·4		0·3							0·2
Spasticity		5·7	6·5		1·9	2·9	1·5	2·5	4·2	1·6	2·6	2·4	2·0	2·6	3·6		3·4		2·5
Short-term memory		5·7												0·3					
Stammer													0·3						
Tongue-tied													0·3						
Thyroid deficiency																			
Visual problems		5·7	9·7	4·4	1·9	3·6	5·9	5·6	2·8	2·8	2·6	3·9	3·5	2·6	6·7	2·8			3·8
Blind (total)		2·9	3·2			2·2			0·4	0·3			0·3						0·3
Colour blind																			
Retinitis pigmentosa													0·3						
Unspecified										0·3	0·9	0·3	0·3						0·4

BIBLIOGRAPHY

Abberton, E., Parker, A. and Fourcin, A. (1977). Speech improvement in deaf adults using laryngograph displays. In *Research Conference on Speech-Processing Aids for the Deaf*. Washington, D.C.

Acts of Parliament: 56 & 57 Victoria, c.42, Elementary Education (Blind and Deaf Children) Act 1893. 7 & 8 George VI, c.31, Education Act 1944.

Agricola, R.P. (1557). *De Inventione Dialectica*.

Albright, M.A. (1944). Ear, eye or both. *Volta Review*, **46**, 11–13.

Amman, J.C. (1700). *A Dissertation on Speech*. Translated by C. Baker, 1873. Low, Marston, Low and Searle, London.

Ando, K. and Canter, G.J. (1969). A study of syllabic stress in some English words as produced by deaf and normally hearing speakers. *Language and Speech*, **12**, 247–55.

Angelocci, A., Kopp, G. and Holbrook, A. (1964). The vowel formants of deaf and normal hearing eleven- to fourteen-year-old boys. *Journal of Speech and Hearing Disorders*, **29**, 156–70.

Aristotle, The Works of. Translated into English (eds J.A. Smith and W.D. Ross, 1910). Clarendon Press, Oxford.

Arnold, T. (1888). *Education of Deaf Mutes*. Werthimer Lea, London.

Augustine, St. *Horesis Pelagianea defensorum*, Liber Tertius, Caput IV-10. Excudebatur et venit apud J.P. Migne, Editorum, 1865.

Ballantyne, J. (1970). Iatrogenic deafness. 16th James Yearsley Memorial Lecture. *Journal of Laryngology*, October, 967–1000.

Barr, B. and Wedenberg, E. (1965). Prognosis of perceptive hearing loss in children with respect to genesis and use of hearing aid. *Acta Otolaryngologica*, **59**, 464–74.

Bede, The Venerable. *Ecclesiastical History of England* also the *Anglo-Saxon Chronicle* (ed. J.A. Giles, 1849). H.G. Bohn, London.

Bell, A.G. (1872). Visible speech as a means of communicating articulation to deaf mutes. *American Annals of the Deaf*, **17**, 1–21.

Bell, A.G. (1916). *The Mechanism of Speech*. Funk and Wagnalls, New York.

Bellefluer, P.A. and Van Dyke, R.C. (1968). The effects of high gain amplification on children in a residential school of the deaf. *Journal of Speech and Hearing Research*, **11**, 343–7.

Bender, R.E. (1970). *The Conquest of Deafness*. The Press of Western Reserve University, Cleveland, Ohio.

Berger, K.W. (1970). Vowel confusions in speech reading. *Journal of Speech and Hearing*, **5**, 123–8.

Berger, K.W. (1972). *Speechreading: Principles and Methods*. National Educational Press, Baltimore.

Berger, K.W., de Pompei, R.A. and Droder, J.L. (1970). The effect of distance on speechreading. *Ohio Journal of Speech and Hearing*, **5**, 115–22.

Black, J.W. (1971). Speech pathology for the deaf. In *Speech for the Deaf Child: Knowledge and Use* (ed. Leo E. Connor). A.G. Bell Association for the Deaf, Washington, D.C.

Bogle, D. and Ingram, T. (1971). *The Edinburgh Articulation Test.* E. & S. Livingstone, London.

Bonet, J.P. (1620). *Simplification of the Letters of the Alphabet and Methods of Teaching Deaf-Mutes to Speak.* Translated by H.N. Dixon, 1890.

Boone, D.R. (1966). Modification of the voices of deaf children. *Volta Review*, **68**, 686–92.

Boothroyd, A. (1972). Sensory aids research project – Clarke School for the Deaf. In *Speech Communication Ability and Profound Deafness* (ed. G. Fant). A.G. Bell Association for the Deaf.

Boothroyd, A. (1973). Some experiments on the control of voice in the profoundly deaf using a pitch extractor and storage oscilloscope display. *IEEE Transactions in Audiology and Electronics*, **AU-21**, 274–8.

Boothroyd, A. (1980). Recommendations to improve preparation of personnel. In *Speech Assessment and Speech Improvement for the Hearing Impaired* (ed. J.D. Subtelny). A.G. Bell Association for the Deaf, Washington, D.C.

Boothroyd, A. and Cawkwell, S. (1970). Vibrotactile thresholds in pure tone audiometry. *Acta Otolaryngologica*, **69**, 381–7.

Boothroyd, A., Nickerson, R.S. and Stevens, K.N. (1974). Temporal patterns in the speech of the deaf – a study in remedial training (S.A.R.P. 15). Clarke School for the Deaf, Northampton, Mass.

Brannon, J.B. (1961). Speechreading of various speech materials. *Journal of Speech and Hearing Disorders*, **26**, 348–52.

Brannon, J.B. (1964). Visual feedback of glossal motions and its influence on the speech of children. Unpublished dissertation, Northwestern University.

Brannon, J.B. (1966). The speech production and spoken language of the deaf. *Language and Speech*, **9**, 127–36.

Brinskey, R.J. and Sinclair, J. (1966). The importance of low frequency amplification in deaf children. *Audecibel*, **15**, 7–20.

Broadbent, D.E. and Ladefoged, P. (1960). Vowel judgements and adaptation level. *Proceedings of the Royal Society of Medicine*, **151**, 384–99.

Brockman, S.J. (1959). An exploratory investigation of delayed progressive neural hypacusis in children. *Archives of Otolaryngology* (Chicago) **70**, 340.

Brooks, D.M. (1973). Gain requirements of hearing aid users. *Scandinavian Audiology*, **2**, 199–205.

Bruhn, M.E. (1942). Methods of teaching lipreading: a symposium. Lip reading as living language. *Volta Review*, **44**, 636–8.

Bruhn, M.E. (1949). *Mueller-Walle method of lipreading.* The Volta Bureau, Washington.

Bulwer, J.B. (1648). *Philocophus, or the Deafe and Dumbe Man's Friend.* Humphrey Moseley, London.

Burchett, J.H. (1950). *Lip reading.* National Institute for the Deaf, London.

Buxton, D. (1880). *Speech for the Deaf.* Essays, Proceedings and Resolutions of the International Congress on the Education of the Deaf.

Calvert, D.R. (1964). An approach to the study of deaf speech. In *Report of the Proceedings of the International Congress on Education of the Deaf*, 242–5. U.S. Government Printing Office, Washington D.C.

Calvert, D.R. and Silverman, S.R. (1975). *Speech and Deafness.* A.G. Bell Association for the Deaf, Washington D.C.

Carhart, R. (1961). Auditory Training. In *Hearing and Deafness* (eds H. Davis and S.R. Silverman). Holt, Rinehart & Winston, New York.

Carlin, W.T. (1964). Speech of partially-hearing school children. Unpublished thesis, University of Manchester.

Cherry, E.C. (1961). *On Human Communication*. Wiley, New York.

Clark, B.R. (1953). Auditory training of profoundly deaf children. Unpublished thesis, University of Manchester.

Clegg, D.G. (1953). *Pattern for the Listening Eye*. National Institute for the Deaf, London.

Colton, R.H. and Cooker, H.S. (1968). Perceived nasality in the speech of the deaf. *Journal of Speech and Hearing Research*, **11**, 553–9.

Conference of Head Masters of Institutions for the Education of the Deaf and Dumb, Proceedings (1877).

Conrad, R. (1976). Speech quality of deaf children. In *Disorders of Auditory Function II* (ed. S.D.G. Stephens). Academic Press, London.

Conrad, R. (1979). *The Deaf School Child. Language and Cognitive Function*. Harper & Row.

Cornett, R.O. (1964). Cued speech. *American Annals of the Deaf*, **112**, 3–13.

Dale, D.M.C. (1958). The possibility of providing extensive experience for severely and profoundly deaf children by the use of hearing aids. Unpublished thesis, University of Manchester.

Dalgarno, G. (1680). *Didascalocophus or the Deaf and Dumb Mans Tutor*. Oxford.

Darbyshire, J.O. (1976). A study of the use of high power hearing aids by children with marked degrees of deafness and the possibility of deterioration in auditory acuity. *British Journal of Audiology*, **10**, 74–82.

Davis, H. and Silverman, S.R. (1961). *Hearing and Deafness*. Holt, Rinehart and Winston, New York.

Davis, H., Stevens, S.S. and Nichols, R.H. (1974). *Hearing Aids: An Experimental Study of Design Objectives*. Harvard University Press, Cambridge, Mass.

Delattre, P.C., Liberman, A.M. and Cooper, F.S. (1955). Acoustic loci and transitional cues for consonants. *Journal of the Acoustical Society of America*, **27**, 769–73.

Denes, P.B. (1963). On the statistics of spoken English. *Journal of the Acoustical Society of America*, **35**, 892–904.

Denes, P.B. and Pinson, E.N. (1963). *The Speech Chain*. Bell Telephone Laboratories, Murray Hill, N.J.

Department of Education and Science (1964). *The Health of the School Child, 1962 and 1963*. H.M.S.O., London.

Department of Education and Science (1972). *The Health of the School Child, 1969 and 1970*. H.M.S.O., London.

Digby, Sir K. *The Private Memoirs of Sir Kenelme Digby* (1827). Saunders and Otley, London.

DiJonson, A. (1971). *Preschool connected speech inventory*. State Department of Education, Harrisburg.

Douek, E., Fourcin, A., Moore, B. and Clarke G. (1977). A new approach to the cochlear implant. *Proceedings of the Royal Society of Medicine*, **70**, 379–83.

Duffy, J.K. (1967). Audio-visual speech audiometry and a new audio and audio-visual speech perception index. *Maico Audiological Library Series*, **5**, 9.

Erber, N.P. (1971). Auditory and audiovisual reception of words in low-frequency noise by children with impaired hearing. *Journal of Speech and Hearing Research*, **14**, 496–512.

Erber, N.P. (1972). Speech-envelope cues as an acoustic aid to lipreading for profoundly deaf children. *Journal of the Acoustical Society of America*, **51**, 1224–7.

Evans, L. (1960). Factors related to listening and lipreading. *Teacher of the Deaf*, **58**, 417–23.

Evans, L. (1965). Psychological factors related to lipreading. *Teacher of the Deaf*, **63**, 131–6.

Ewing, A.W.G. (1956). The education of the deaf: History of the Department of Education of the Deaf, University of Manchester 1919–1955. *British Journal of Educational Studies*, **4**, 103–28.

Ewing, A.W.G. (1964). *Educational Guidance and the Deaf Child*. Manchester University Press.

Ewing, A.W.G. and Ewing E.C. (1964). *Teaching Deaf Children to Talk*. Manchester University Press.

Ewing, A.W.G., Ewing, I.R. and Littler, T.S. (1936). *The Use of Hearing Aids*. Medical Research Council report.

Ewing, I.R. (1941). Lipreading for adults. *Teacher of the Deaf*, **39**, 3–6.

Ewing, I.R. (1957). Screening tests and guidance clinics for babies and young children. In *Educational Guidance and the Deaf Child* (ed. A.W.G. Ewing). Manchester University Press.

Ewing, I.R. (1967). *Hearing Aids, Lipreading and Deaf Speech*. Manchester University Press.

Ewing, I.R. and Ewing A.W.G. (1938). *The Handicap of Deafness*. Longmans Green, London.

Ewing, I.R. and Ewing A.W.G. (1954). *Speech and the Deaf Child*. Manchester University Press.

Ewing, I.R. and Ewing, A.W.G. (1958). *New Opportunities for Deaf Children*. University of London Press.

Farrar, A. (1923). *Arnold on the Education of the Deaf*. National College of Teachers of the Deaf, London.

Fisher, M.T. (1968). *Improve your Lipreading*. The Volta Review, Washington.

Fitzgerald, A. and Markides, A. (1982). Comparative speech discrimination abilities of hearing-impaired children achieved through the Infra-red and Radio hearing aid systems. *Journal of the British Association of Teachers of the Deaf*, **6**, 10–17.

Fletcher, H. (1929). *Speech and Hearing*. Van Nostrand, New York.

Forner, L.L. and Hixon, T.J. (1977). Respiratory kinematics in profoundly hearing-impaired speakers. *Journal of Speech and Hearing Research*, **20**, 373–407.

Franks, J.R. and Oyer, H.J. (1967). Factors influencing the identification of English sounds in lipreading. *Journal of Speech and Hearing Research*, **10**, 757–64.

Fry, D.B. (1963). Coding and decoding in speech. In *Sign, Signals and Symbols* (ed. S.E. Mason). Methuen, London.

Fry, D.B. (1964). The reception of speech. Chapter IV in *The Deaf Child* by Whetnall and Fry. William Heinemann Medical Books.

Fry, D.B. (1977). *Homo Loquens – Man as a Talking Animal*. Cambridge University Press.

Gallaudet, E.M. (1874). Results of articulation teaching at Northampton. *American Annals of the Deaf and Dumb*, **19**, 136–45.

Gallaudet, E.M. (1910). *Life of Thomas Hopkins Gallaudet*. Henry Holt, New York.

Gault, R.H. (1926). The interpretation of speech by tactual and visual impressions. *Archives of Otolaryngology*, **3**, 228–39.

Gault, R.H. (1927). On the identification of certain vowel and consonantal elements in words by their tactual qualities and by their visual qualities as seen by the lipreader. *Journal of Abnormal Psychology*, **22**, 33–9.

Gault, R.H. (1928). Interpretation of spoken language when the feel of speech supplements vision on the speaking face. *Volta Review*, **30**, 379–86.

Geffner, D. and Freeman, L.R. (1980). Speech assessment at the primary level: Interpretation relative to speech training. In *Speech Assessment and Speech Improvement for the Hearing Impaired* (ed.J.D. Subtelny). A.G. Bell Association for the Deaf, Washington D.C.

Gengel, R. (1974). Discussion: Aided speech reception of hearing-impaired children, perceptual and cognitive strategies. In *Sensory Capabilities of Hearing Impaired Children* (ed. R.E. Stark). University Park Press.

Gentleman's Magazine (1807) London.

Gessel, A. (1940). *The First Five Years of Life*. Methuen, London.

Goldman, R. and Fristoe, M. (1972). *Goldman–Fristoe Test of Articulation*. American Guidance Service, Circle Pines, Minn.

Goldstein, M.A. (1939). *The Acoustic Method for Training of the Deaf and Hard-of-hearing Child*. The Laryngoscope Press, St Louis.

Green, F. (1783). *Vox Oculis Subjecta: A Dissertation on the Most Curious and Important Art of Imparting Speech and the Knowledge of Language, to the Naturally Deaf, and (consequently) dumb; with a particular account of the Academy of Messrs Braidwood of Edinburgh*. B. White, London.

Griffiths, R. (1954). *The Abilities of Babies*. University of London Press.

Gulian, E. and Hinds, P. (1980). Response bias in the perception of deaf speech by experienced and naive listeners. *British Journal of Audiology*, **15**, 165–71.

Hamp, E.P. (1957). *A Glossary of American Technical Linguistic Usage, 1925–1950*. Spectrum, Utrecht and Antwerp.

Hardy, W.G., Pauls, M.D. and Haskins, H.L. (1958). An analysis of language development in children with impaired hearing. *Acta Otolaryngologica* (Suppl. 141).

Harris, K.S. (1958). Cues for the discrimination of American English fricatives in spoken syllables. *Language and Speech*, **1**, 1–7.

Haycock, G.S. (1933). *The Teaching of Speech*. The Volta Review, Washington D.C.

Heider, F.K. and Heider, G.M. (1940). An experimental investigation of lipreading. *Psychological Monographs*, **52**, 124–33.

Heidinger, V.A. (1972). An exploratory study of procedures for improving temporal features in the speech of deaf children. Unpublished dissertation, Columbia University (quoted by Ling, 1976).

Heinicke, S. (1790). *Neues A.B.C. Sylben und Lesebugh*. Leipzig.

Hine, W.D. and Furness, H.J.S. (1975). Does wearing a hearing aid damage residual hearing? *Teacher of the Deaf*, **73**, 261–71.

Hirsh, I.J. (1965). Perception of speech. In *Sensorineural Hearing Processes and Disorders* (ed. A.B. Brown). International Symposium, Henry Ford Hospital, USA.

Hixon, T.J., Saxman, J.H. and McQueen, H.D. (1967). A respirometric technique for evaluating velopharyngeal competence during speech. *Folia Phoniatrica*, **19**, 203–19.

Hodgson, K.W. (1953). *The Deaf and their Problems*. Watts, London.

Hoffman, H.S. (1958). Study of some cues in the perception of the voiced stop consonants. *Journal of the Acoustical Society of America*, **30**, 1035–41.

Holder, W. (1669). *Elements of Speech with an Appendix concerning Persons Deaf and Dumb*. J. Martyn, London.

Holm, C. (1970). Oral presentation at the First International Colloquium on the Verbotonal System. Primosten (Yugoslavia), January 29–31.

Holmgren, L. (1940). Can the hearing be damaged by a hearing aid? *Acta Otolaryngologica*, **28**, 440.

Hood, R.B. (1966). Some physical concomitants of the perception of speech rhythm of the deaf. PhD thesis abstract. Stanford University, California.

Hood, R.B. and Dixon, R.F. (1949). Physical characteristics of speech rhythm of deaf and normal-hearing speakers. *Journal of Communication Disorders*, **2**, 20–8.

Hopkins, L.A. (1953). The relationship between degrees of deafness and response to acoustic training. *Volta Review*, **55**, 23.

Houde, R.A. (1980). Evaluation of independent drill with visual aids for speech training. In *Speech Assessment and Speech Improvement for the Hearing Impaired* (ed. J.D. Subtelny). A.G. Bell Association for the Deaf, Washington D.C.

Hudgins, C.V. (1934). A comparative study of the speech coordinations of deaf and normal subjects. *Journal of Genetic Psychology*, **44**, 1–48.

Hudgins, C.V. (1946). Speech breathing and speech intelligibility. *Volta Review*, **48**, 642–7.

Hudgins, C.V. (1949). A method of appraising the speech of the deaf. *Volta Review*, **46**, 597–601.

Hudgins, C.V. (1954). Auditory training: its possibilities and limitations. *Volta Review*, **56**, 1.

Hudgins, C.V., Marquis, R.J., Nichols, R.H., Peterson, G.E. and Ross, D.A. (1948). The comparative performance of an experimental hearing aid and two commercial instruments. *Journal of the Acoustical Society of America*, **20**, 241–58.

Hudgins, C.V. and Numbers, F. (1942). An investigation of the intelligibility of the speech of the deaf. *Genetic Psychology Monographs*, **25**, 289–392.

Huggins, A.W.F. (1972). On the perception of temporal phenomena in speech. *Journal of the Acoustical Society of America*, **51**, 1279–90.

Hughes, G. and Halle, M. (1956). Spectral properties of fricative consonants. *Journal of the Acoustical Society of America*, **28**, 303–10.

Hughson, W., Ciocco, A. and Palmer, C. (1939). An audiometric study of pupils in the Pennsylvania School for the Deaf. *Archives of Otolaryngology*, **29**, 403.

Hughson, W., Ciocco, A., Whitting, G.E. and Lawrence, S.P. (1941). An analysis of speech characteristics in deafened children with observation on training method. *The Laryngoscope*, **51**, 868–91.

Huizing, H.C. (1959). Deaf mutism: Modern trends in treatment and prevention. *Annals Oto-Rhino-Laryngology*, **5**, 74–106.

Hutchinson, J.M., Kornhauser, R.L., Beasley, D.S. and Beasley, D.C. (1978). Aerodynamic functioning in consonant production in hearing-impaired children. *Audiology, Hearing, Education*, **4**, 23–31.

Hutchinson, J.M. and Smith, L.L. (1976). Aerodynamic functioning during consonant production by hearing-impaired adults. *Audiology, Hearing, Education,* **2,** 16–24.

Hutchinson, J.M. and Smith, L.L. (1980). Language and speech of the hearing impaired. In *Introduction to Aural Rehabilitation* (eds R.L. Schow and M.A. Nerbonne). University Park Press, Baltimore.

Hutton, C. (1959). Combining auditory and visual stimuli in aural rehabilitation. *Volta Review,* **61,** 316–19.

Illingworth, R.S. (1960). *The Development of the Infant and Young Child.* E. & S. Livingstone, Edinburgh.

Irwin, R.B. (1974). Evaluating the perception and articulation of phonemes of children, ages 5–8. *Journal of Communication Disorders,* **7,** 45–63.

Jensema, C., Karchmer, M. and Trybus, R. (1978). *The rated speech intelligibility of hearing-impaired children.* Office of Demographic Studies, Gallaudet College, Washington D.C.

Jensema, C. and Trybus, R. (1978). *Communication patterns and educational achievement of hearing-impaired students.* Office of Demographic Studies, Gallaudet College, Washington D.C.

John, J.E.J. (1957). Acoustics in the use of hearing aids. In *Educational Guidance and the Deaf Child* (ed. A.W.G. Ewing). Manchester University Press.

John, J.E.J. (1975). The linguistic input to a hearing aid. Paper presented at the second conference of the British Society of Audiology, Southampton.

John, J.E.J., Gemmill, J., Howarth, J., Kitzinger, M. and Sykes, M. (1976). Some factors affecting the intelligibility of deaf children's speech. In *Disorders of Auditory Function II* (ed. S.D.G. Stephens). Academic Press, London.

John, J.E.J. and Howarth, J.N. (1965). The effect of time distortions on the intelligibility of deaf children's speech. *Language and Speech,* **8,** 127–34.

Johnson, E.H. (1939). Testing results of acoustic training. *American Annals of the Deaf,* **84,** 223–33.

Johnson, J.C. (1962). *Educating Hearing-Impaired Children in Ordinary Schools.* Manchester University Press.

Karchmer, M., Allen, T., Petersen, L. and Quaynor, A. (1982). Hearing-impaired children and youth in Canada. Student characteristics in relation to manual communication patterns in four special education settings. *American Annals of the Deaf,* **127,** 89–104.

Karchmer, M., Milone, M. and Wolk, S. (1979). Educational significance of hearing loss at three levels of severity. *American Annals of the Deaf,* **124,** 97–109.

Karchmer, M. and Trybus, R.J. (1977). *Who are the deaf children in 'mainstream' programs?* Office of Demographic Studies, Gallaudet College, Washington D.C.

Karchmer, M., Trybus, R.J. and Paquin, M. (1978). Early manual communication, parental hearing status, and the academic achievement of deaf students. Paper presented to the Am-Ed. Res. Assoc. Toronto.

Kerr Love, J. (1893). *Papers on Deaf-Mutism.* Glasgow.

Kerr Love, J. and Addison, W.H. (1896). *Deaf Mutism.* Madehose, Glasgow.

Kinney, C.E. (1953). Hearing impairments in children. *Laryngoscope,* **63,** 220–6.

Kinney, C.E. (1961). The further destruction of partially deafened children's hearing by the use of powerful hearing aids. *Annals of Otology,* **70,** 828–35.

Kinzie, C.E. and Kinzie, R. (1931). *Lip-reading for the Deafened Adult*. John C. Winston, Philadelphia.

Kozhevnikov, V.A. and Christovich, L.A. (1965). *Speech: Articulation and Perception*. English Translation J.P.R.S., Washington D.C. No. JPRS 30543.

Kröhnert, O. (1966). *Die Sprachliche Bildung des Gehörlosen*. Beltz, Weinheim.

Kroiss, K. (1903). *Zur Methodik des Hörunterichts*. Berguian, Wiesbaden.

Kyle, J.G. (1977). Audiometric analysis as a predictor of speech intelligibility. *British Journal of Audiology*, **11,** 51–8.

Kyle, J.G., Conrad, R., McKenzie, M.G., Morris, A.J.M. and Weiskrantz, B.C. (1978). Language abilities in deaf school leavers. *Journal of the British Association of Teachers of the Deaf*, **2,** 38–42.

Larr, A.L. (1959). Speechreading through closed circuit television. *Volta Review*, **61,** 19–22.

Lasso, el Licenciado (1550). *Tratado legal sobre los mudós*. Biblioteca Nacional, Madrid.

Lehiste, I. (1970). *Suprasegmentals*. The M.I.T. Press, Cambridge, Mass. and London.

l'Epée, C.M. de (1784). *La Véritable Manière d'Instruire les Sourds et Muets*. Chez Nyon l'Aine, Paris.

Levitt, H. (1971). Speech production and the deaf child. In *Speech for the Deaf Child: Knowledge and Use* (ed. Lco E. Connor). A.G. Bell Association for the Deaf, Washington D.C.

Levitt, H. (1980). Speech assessment: Intermediate and secondary levels. In *Speech Assessment and Speech Improvement for the Hearing Impaired* (ed. J.D. Subtelny). A.G. Bell Association for the Deaf, Washington D.C.

Levitt, H., Pickett, J.M. and Houde, R. (1980). *Sensory Aids for the Hearing-Impaired*. IEEE Press, New York.

Levitt, H., Smith, C. and Strombert, H. (1974). Acoustic perceptual and articulatory characteristics of the speech of deaf children. Speech Communication Seminar, Stockholm.

Levitt, H., Stark, R.E., McGarr, N., Carp, J., Strombert, M., Gaffney, R.H., Barry, C., Vilez, A., Osverger, M.J., Leiter, E. and Freeman, L. (1976). *Proceedings of Language Assessment for the Hearing Impaired. A work-study institute*. New York State Education Department, New York State School for the Deaf.

Lewis, M.M. (1951). *Infant Speech. A Study of the Beginnings of Language*. Routledge and Kegan Paul, London.

Liberman, A.M., Delattre, P. and Cooper, F.S. (1952). The role of selected stimuli variables in the perception of unvoiced stop consonants. *American Journal of Psychology*, **65,** 487–503.

Ling, D. (1964). Implications of hearing aid amplification below 300 cps. *Volta Review*, **66,** 723–9.

Ling, D. (1976). *Speech and the Hearing-Impaired Child: Theory and Practice*, A.G. Bell Association for the Deaf, Washington D.C.

Ling, D. (1979). Four experiments on speech. *Blue Window*, Gallaudet College, Washington, D.C.

Ling, D. and Milne, M. (1979). The development of speech in hearing-impaired children. In *Proceedings of the International Symposium on Amplification in Education*. A.G. Bell Association, Washington D.C.

Löwe, A. (1980). The historical development of oral education. In *Oral*

Education Today and Tomorrow (ed. A.M. Mulholland). A.G. Bell Association for the Deaf, Washington D.C.

McCandless, G.A. (1976). Special consideration in evaluating children and the aging for hearing aids. In *Hearing Aids: Current Developments and Concepts.* University Park Press, Baltimore.

McCarthy, D. (1970). Language development in children. In *Carmichael's Manual of Child Psychology* (ed. P.H. Mussen) 3rd edn. John Wiley, New York.

McCormick, B. (1980). The assessment of audio-visual and visual speech discrimination skills in aural rehabilitation programmes. In *Disorders of Auditory Function III* (eds I.G. Taylor and A. Markides). Academic Press, London.

McGarr, N.S. (1980). Evaluation of speech in intermediate school-aged deaf children. In *Speech Assessment and Speech Improvement for the Hearing Impaired* (ed. J.D. Subtelny). A.G. Bell Association for the Deaf, Washington D.C.

McMahon, M.A. and Subtelny, D. (1981). Simultaneous listening, reading, and speaking for improvement of speech. *Volta Review,* **83,** 206–14.

McPherson, D.L. and Davis, M.S. (1978). *Advances in Prosthetic Devices for the Deaf: A technical workshop.* National Technical Institute for the Deaf, Rochester N.Y.

Macrae, J.H. (1967). TTS and recovery from TTS after use of powerful hearing aids. *Journal of the Acoustical Society of America,* **43,** 1445–6.

Macrae, J.H. (1968). Deterioration of the residual hearing of children with sensori-neural deafness. *Acta Otolaryngologica,* **66,** 33–9.

Macrae, J.H. and Farrant, R.H. (1965). The effect of hearing aid use on the residual hearing of children with sensorineural deafness. *Annals of Otology,* **74,** 409–19.

Mangan, K. (1961). Speech improvement through articulation testing. *American Annals of the Deaf,* **106,** 391–6.

Markides, A. (1967). The speech of deaf and partially-hearing children with special reference to factors affecting intelligibility. Unpublished thesis, University of Manchester.

Markides, A. (1971). Do hearing aids damage the user's residual hearing? *Sound* (now *British Journal of Audiology*), **5,** 22–31.

Markides, A. (1976). The effect of hearing aid use on the user's residual hearing. *Scandinavian Audiology,* **5,** 205–10.

Markides, A. (1977). *Binaural Hearing Aids.* Academic Press, London and New York.

Markides, A. (1978). Assessing the speech intelligibility of hearing-impaired children. Oral reading versus picture description. *Journal of the British Association of Teachers of the Deaf,* **2,** 185–9.

Markides, A. (1980a). Type of pure tone audiogram configuration and speech intelligibility. *Journal of the British Association of Teachers of the Deaf,* **4,** 125–9.

Markides, A. (1980b). Type of pure tone audiogram configuration and misarticulations. *Journal of the British Association of Teachers of the Deaf,* **4,** 156–65.

Markides, A. (1980c). Best listening levels of hearing-impaired children. *Journal of the British Association of Teachers of the Deaf,* **4,** 190–7.

Markides, A. (1980*d*). The Manchester speechreading (lipreading) test. In *Disorders of Auditory Function III* (eds I.G. Taylor and A. Markides). Academic Press, London.

Markides, A. (in preparation *a*). The uses and abuses of individual hearing aids in schools.

Markides, A. (in preparation *b*). Uses and abuses of group hearing aids.

Markides, A. and Aryee, D.T.-K. (1978). The effect of hearing aid use on the user's residual hearing – A follow-up study. *Scandinavian Audiology*, **7**, 19–23.

Markides, A. and Aryee, D.T.-K. (1980). The effect of hearing aid use on the user's residual hearing. *Scandinavian Audiology*, **9**, 55–8.

Markides, A., Huntington, A. and Kettlety, A. (1980). Comparative speech discrimination abilities of hearing-impaired children achieved through infra-red, radio and conventional hearing aids. *Journal of the British Association of Teachers of the Deaf*, **4**, 5–14.

Martin, M.C. (1973). Hearing aid gain requirements in sensori-neural hearing loss. *British Journal of Audiology*, **7**, 21–4.

Martin, M.C. (1979). Personal communication.

Martin, M.C., Brooks, D. and Morris, T. (1977). Listening levels through hearing aids: a difference of opinion. *Scandinavian Audiology*, **6**, 107–13.

Martin, M.C. and Lodge, J.J. (1969). A survey of hearing aids in schools for the deaf and partially hearing units. *Sound*, **3**, 2–11.

Mártony, J. (1968). On the correction of voice pitch level for severely hard of hearing subjects. *American Annals of the Deaf*, **113**, 195–202.

Mason, M.K. and Bright, M. (1937). Tempo in rhythmic speech education. *American Annals of the Deaf*, **82**, 385–401.

Medical Research Council (1947). *Hearing aids and audiometers*. Special Report Series No. 261, H.M.S.O., London.

Miller, G.A. (1951). *Language and Communication*. McGraw-Hill, New York.

Miller, G.A., Heise, C.A. and Lichten, D. (1951). The intelligibility of speech as a function of the context of the test material. *Journal of Experimental Psychology*, **41**, 329–35.

Miller-Shaw, M.O. (1936). A study in the analysis and correction of the speech of the hard of hearing. *American Annals of the Deaf*, **81**, 225–31.

Mineter, K. (1982). Assessing the speech intelligibility of hearing-impaired children: Auditory versus audio-visual approach. M.Ed. thesis, University of Manchester.

Møller, T.T. and Rojskjaer, C. (1960). Injury to hearing through hearing aid treatment (acoustic trauma). Fifth Congress, International Society of Audiology, Bonn.

Monsen, R.B. (1974). Durational aspects of vowel production in the speech of deaf children. *Journal of Speech and Hearing Research*, **17**, 386–98.

Monsen, R.B. (1976). The production of English stop consonants in the speech of deaf children. *Journal of Phonetics*, **4**, 29–41.

Monsen, R.B. (1978). Towards measuring how well hearing-impaired children speak. *Journal of Speech and Hearing Research*, **21**, 197–219.

Morris, D.M. (1944). A study of some of the factors involved in lipreading. M.A. thesis, Smith College.

Morris, T. (1975). A guide to selecting gain settings for children suffering severe congenital sensori-neural deafness. Occasional paper No. 1 Royal School for the Deaf, Manchester.

Murphy, K.P. (1957). Tests of abilities and attainments. Pupils in schools for the deaf aged twelve. In *Educational Guidance and the Deaf Child* (ed. A.W.G. Ewing). Manchester University Press.

Murray, N.E. (1951). *Hearing aids and classification of deaf children*. Report CAL-IR-2, Commonwealth Acoustic Laboratories, Sydney (quoted by Macrae and Farrant).

Myklebust, H.R. (1960). *The Psychology of Deafness*. Grune and Stratton, New York.

Nabelek, A.K. (1980). Effects of room acoustics on speech perception through hearing aids. In *Binaural Hearing and Amplification I*. (ed. E. Robert Libby). Zenetron, Chicago.

Nabelek, A.K. and Pickett, J.M. (1974). Reception of consonants in a classroom as affected by monaural and binaural listening, noise, reverberation and hearing aids. *Journal of the Acoustical Society of America*, **56**, 628–39.

Naunton, R.F. (1957). The effect of hearing aid use upon the user's residual hearing. *Laryngoscope*, **67**, 569–76.

Navarro-Tomas, T. (1920). *Juan Pablo Bonet*. Imprenta de la Casa de Curitat, Barcelona.

Navarro-Tomas, T. (1924). Manuel Ramirez de Cárrion y el art de ensenar a hablar a los mudos. *Revista de filologia española*, **11**, 225–30.

Nickerson, R.S. (1973). *Computerized speech-training aids for the deaf*. Report No. 2366: Bolt, Beraneck and Newman.

Nitchie, E.B. (1912). *Lipreading, Principles and Practices*. F. Stokes, New York.

Nitchie, E.B. (1915). The use of homophenous words. *Volta Review*, **18**, 3.

Nober, E.H. (1967). Articulation of the deaf. *Exceptional Child*, **33**, 611–21.

Numbers, M.E. and Hudgins, C.V. (1948). Speech perception in present day education for deaf children. *Volta Review*, **50**, 449–56.

O'Connor, J.C., Liberman, A.M., Delattre, P.C. and Cooper, F.S. (1957). Acoustic cues for the perception of initial /w, j, r, l/ in English. *Word*, **13**, 24–9.

Olsen, W.O. and Carhart, R. (1967). Development and test procedures for evaluation of binaural hearing aids. *Bulletin of Prosthetics Research*, **10**, 22–49.

O'Neill, J.J. (1951). An exploratory investigation of lip-reading ability among normal-hearing students. *Speech Monographs*, **18**, 309–11.

O'Neill, J.J. (1954). Contributions of the visual components of oral symbols to speech comprehension. *Journal of Speech and Hearing Disorders*, **19**, 429–39.

O'Neill, J.J. and Oyer, H.J. (1961). *Visual Communication for the Hard of Hearing*. Prentice Hall, Englewood Cliffs N.J.

Overbeck, J.C. (1960). Response to speech and music. In *The Modern Educational Treatment of Deafness* (ed. A.W.G. Ewing). The Volta Review, Washington D.C.

Pendergast, K., Dickey, S.E., Selmar, J.W. and Sodir, A.L. (1969). *The Photo Articulation Test*. Interstate Printers and Publishers.

Penn, J.P. (1955). Voice and speech patterns of the hard-of-hearing. *Acta Otolaryngologica* (Suppl. 124).

Pickett, J.M. (1963). Tactual communication of speech sounds to the deaf: Comparison with lipreading. *Journal of Speech and Hearing Disorders*, **28**, 315–30.

Pickett, J.M. (1977). Speech processing aids for the deaf. Proceedings of a conference held at Gallaudet College, Washington D.C.

Pickett, J.M. (1981). Speech, technology and communication for the hearing-impaired. *Volta Review*, **83**, 301–9.

Pitman, J. (1962). Teaching the deaf. *Teacher of the Deaf*, **60**, 311–16.

Plato. *Cratylus, Phaedo, Parmenides* and *Timaeus of Platee*. Translated by Thomas Taylor 1973. Benjamin and John White, London.

Pollack, D. (1964). Acoupedics: a uni-sensory approach to auditory training. *Volta Review*, **66**, 400–9.

Powell, C.A. and Tucker, I.G. (1976). A method of predicting the optimum listening levels of hearing-impaired children. *Scandinavian Audiology*, **5**, 167–76.

Prall, J. (1957). Lipreading and hearing aids combine for better information. *Volta Review*, **59**, 64–5.

Pritchard, D.G. (1970). *Education and the Handicapped*. Routledge & Kegan Paul, New York.

Rawlings, C.G. (1936). A comparative study of the movements of the breathing muscles in speech and in quiet breathing of deaf and normal subjects. *American Annals of the Deaf*, **81**, 136–50.

Redgate, W.G. (1964). Diagnostic tests of reading ability. Unpublished thesis, University of Manchester.

Reuschert, E. (1905). *Friedrich Moritz Hill, der Reformator des deutschen Taubstummenunterrichts*. Dude, Berlin.

Rice, C.G. (1965). Hearing aid design criteria. *International Audiology*, **4**, 130–4.

Risberg, A. (1968). Visual aids for speech correction. *American Annals of the Deaf*, **113**, 178–94.

Roberts, C. (1970). Can hearing aids damage hearing? *Acta Otolaryngologica*, **69**, 123–5.

Ross, M. and Lerman, J. (1967). Hearing aid usage and its effect on residual hearing: a review of the literature and an investigation. *Archives of Otolaryngology*, **86**, 639–44.

Ross, M. and Truex, H. (1965). Protecting residual hearing in hearing aid users. *Archives of Otolaryngology*, **82**, 615–17.

Royal Commission on the Blind, the Deaf and Dumb and Others of the United Kingdom, Report (1889). H.M.S.O.

Sanders, D.A. (1961). A follow-up study of fifty deaf children who received pre-school training. Unpublished thesis, University of Manchester.

Sarrail, S. (1951). Basic percentage of error in lip reading. *Otolaryngology* (Buenos Aires), **2**, 271–7.

Sataloff, J. (1961). Pitfalls in routine hearing testing. *Archives of Otolaryngology*, **73**, 717–26.

Schwartz, J.R. and Black, J.W. (1967). Some effects of sentence structure on speech reading. *Central States Speech Journal*, **18**, 86–90.

Scuri, D. (1935). Respirazione e fonazione nei sordomuti. *Rassegna di sordomuti e fonetica biologica*, **14**, 82–113.

Shannon, C.E. (1949). A mathematical theory of communication. *Bell System Technical Journal*, **27**, 379–423, 623–56.

Sheridan, M.D. (1948). *The Child's Hearing for Speech*. Methuen, London.

Smith, C.R. (1973). *Residual hearing and speech production in deaf children*. Communications Science Laboratory Research Report No. 4, City University of New York.

Smith, C.R. (1975). Residual hearing and speech production in deaf children. *Journal of Speech and Hearing Research*, **18**, 795–811.

Smith, C.R. (1980). Speech assessment at the elementary level: Interpretation relative to speech training. In *Speech Assessment and Speech Improvement for the Hearing Impaired* (ed. J.D. Subtelny). A.G. Bell Association for the Deaf, Washington, D.C.

Society for Training Teachers of the Deaf and Diffusion of the German System. Prospectus of the Society (1878). London.

Stark, R. and Levitt, H. (1974). Prosodic features reception and production in deaf children. *Journal of the Acoustical Society of America*, **55**, 163.

Stevens, K.N. and House, A.S. (1955). Development of a quantitative description of vowel articulation. *Journal of the Acoustical Society of America*, **27**, 484–93.

Stevens, P. (1960). Spectre of fricative noise in human speech. *Language and Speech*, **3**, 32–49.

Story, A.J. (1901). *Speech for the Deaf*. Hill and Ainsworth, Stoke on Trent.

Story, A.J. (1915). *Speech, Reading and Speech for the Deaf*. Hill and Ainsworth, Stoke on Trent.

Stratton, W. (1974). Intonation feedback for the deaf through a tactile display. *Volta Review*, **76**, 26–35.

Strong, W. (1975). Speech aids for the profoundly/severely hearing impaired. *Volta Review*, **77**, 536–56.

Taaffe, G. and Wong, W. (1957). Studies of variables in lip reading stimulus materials. John Tracy Clinic Research Papers III.

Templin, M.O. and Darley, F.L. (1969). *The Templin–Darley Tests of Articulation*. Bureau of Education Research and Service, University of Iowa.

Thomas, W. (1963). Intelligibility of the speech of deaf children. *Proceedings of International Congress on the Education of the Deaf*. Document No. 106.

Tillman, T.W., Carhart, R. and Olsen, W.O. (1970). Hearing aid efficiency in a competing speech situation. *Journal of Speech and Hearing Research*, **13**, 789–811.

Tong, Y.C., Clark, G.M., Seligman, P.M. and Patrick, J.F. (1980). Speech processing for a multiple-electrode cochlear implant hearing prosthesis. *Journal of the Acoustical Society of America*, **68**, 1897–9.

Trybus, R.J. (1980). National data on rated speech intelligibility of hearing-impaired children. In *Speech Assessment and Speech Improvement for the Hearing Impaired* (ed. J.D. Subtelny). A.G. Bell Association for the Deaf, Washington, D.C.

Upton, H.W. (1968). Wearable eyeglass speechreading aid. *American Annals of the Deaf*, **113**, 222–9.

van Praagh, W. (1878). *On the Oral Education of the Deaf and Dumb*. Journal of Education. Association for the Oral Instruction of the Deaf, London.

van Praagh, W. (1884). *Lessons for the Instruction of Deaf and Dumb Children*. Truebner, London.

van Uden, A. (1960). A sound-perceptive method. In *The Modern Educational Treatment of Deafness* (ed. A.W.G. Ewing). The Volta Review, Washington.

van Uden, A. (1970). New realisations in the light of the pure oral method. *Volta Review*, **72**, 524–37.

Vatter, J. (1875). *Der verbundene Sach-und Sprachunterricht*. Bechhold, Frankfurt.

Vernon, M. and Mindel, E.D. (1971). Psychological and psychiatric aspects of profound hearing loss. In *Audiological Assessment* (ed. D.E. Rose), Prentice-Hall, Englewood Cliffs, N.J.

Voelker, A.C. (1935). A preliminary strobophotoscopic study of the speech of the deaf. *American Annals of the Deaf*, **80**, 243–7.

Voelker, A.C. (1938). An experimental study of the comparative rate of utterance of deaf and normal speakers. *American Annals of the Deaf*, **83**, 274–83.

Wallis, J. (1653). *De Loquella Sive Sonorum Foratione Tractatus Grammatico-Physicus*. Editio Sexta. Lugduni, Batavorum: Apud Jo. Arm. Langerak.

Wallis, J. (1678). *A Defence of the Royal Society, In Answer to the Cavils of Dr. Holder*. Supplement to the Philosophical Transactions of the Royal Society.

Warnock, H.M. (1979). *Special Educational Needs*. Report of the Committee of Enquiry into the Education of Handicapped Children and Young People. H.M.S.O., London.

Watson, J. (1809). *Instruction of the Deaf and Dumb*. Darton and Harvey, London.

Watson, T.J. (1952). Dr James Kerr Love. *Teacher of the Deaf*, **50**, 7.

Watson, T.J. (1956). The use of hearing aids with severely deaf children. *Archives of Otolaryngology*, **64**, 151–6.

Watson, T.J. (1964). The use of hearing aids by hearing-impaired children in ordinary schools. *Volta Review*, **66**, 741.

Watson, T.J. (1967). *The Education of Hearing-handicapped Children*. University of London Press.

Watson, T.J. (1980). Reaction to 'The historical development of oral education'. In *Oral Education Today and Tomorrow* (ed. A.M. Mulholland). A.G. Bell Association for the Deaf, Washington D.C.

Watts, A.F. (1960). *The Language and Mental Development of Children*. Harrap, London.

Wedenberg, E. (1951). Auditory training of deaf and hard of hearing children. *Acta Otolaryngologica*, **94**, 130.

Wedenberg, E. (1954). Auditory training of severely hard of hearing pre-school children. *Acta Otolaryngologica*, Supplement 110.

Werner, H. (1932). *History of the Problem of Deaf-mutism until the 17th Century*. (Translated from the original German text by C.K. Bonning).

Whetnall, E. (1964). Binaural hearing. *Journal of Laryngology and Otology*, **78**, 1079–89.

Whetnall, E. and Fry, D.B. (1964). *The Deaf Child*, William Heinemann Medical Books.

Whitton, H. (1956). Sir James E. Jones: Benefactor to the deaf. *Teacher of the Deaf*, **54**, 66–70.

Wollman, D.C. (1961). Some problems involved in the application of secondary modern education for deaf pupils with special reference to the institution of a leaving certificate. Unpublished thesis, University of Manchester.

Wood, K.S. and Blakely, R.W. (1953). The association of lipreading and the ability to understand distorted speech. *Western Speech*, **17**, 259–61.

Woodward, M.F. and Lowell, E.E. (1964). *A linguistic approach to the education of aurally-handicapped children*. United States Department of Health, Education and Welfare Project 907.

Worcester, A.E. (1915). Pronunciation of sight. *Volta Review*, **17**, 85–93.

World Health Organisation (1967). *The early detection and treatment of handicapping defects in young children.* Special Report distributed by Regional Office for Europe, Copenhagen.

Wright, H.N. and Carhart, R. (1960). The efficiency of binaural hearing among the hearing impaired. *AMA Archives of Otolaryngology*, **72,** 789–97.

AUTHOR INDEX

SUBJECT INDEX